THE ESSENTIAL
OVER 35
PREGNANCY
GUIDE

THE ESSENTIAL OVER 35 PREGNANCY GUIDE

EVERYTHING YOU NEED TO KNOW ABOUT BECOMING A MOTHER LATER IN LIFE

ELLEN ROSE LAVIN, PH.D.

WITH SAMUEL H. WOOD, M.D.

AVON BOOKS ◆ NEW YORK

All women, pregnant or otherwise, are strongly advised to consult with their medical caregivers before taking any medications or starting any diet or exercise programs. The author and publisher disclaim any liability arising directly or indirectly from the use of this book.

AVON BOOKS
A division of
The Hearst Corporation
1350 Avenue of the Americas
New York, New York 10019

Copyright © 1998 by Ellen Rose Lavin
Published by arrangement with the author
Visit our website at http://www.AvonBooks.com
ISBN: 0-380-78819-5

Library of Congress Cataloging in Publication Data:
Lavin, Ellen Rose.
    The essential over 35 pregnancy guide : everything you need to know about becoming a mother later in life / Ellen Rose Lavin.
        p.   cm.
    Includes bibliographical references and index.
    1. Pregnancy in middle age—Popular works.   I. Title.
RG556.6.L38   1998
618.2'4—dc21   97-37542
                                                                                      CIP

First Avon Books Printing: April 1998

AVON TRADEMARK REG. U.S. PAT. OFF. AND IN OTHER COUNTRIES, MARCA REGISTRADA, HECHO EN U.S.A.

Printed in the U.S.A.

OPM   10   9   8   7   6   5   4   3   2   1

DEDICATION

To Rick, for all the obvious reasons

CONTENTS

PART TWO: BEING PREGNANT

PREFACE

I became a mother at 41. *Now* I know how much it matters to be someone's mother, but if it's true that our natural interests and innate leanings as children forecast what *will* matter to us someday, then the fulfillment of my heart's desire later as an adult—having a baby—turned out to be something of a surprise.

When I was a little girl, I wasn't a full-fledged tomboy, but neither did I play much with dolls. I guess you could say that in this regard, I was "in-between." Outside of playing with my three-foot-tall Dance-With-Me doll—the kind with straps on the feet you slip yours into so you can hop and twirl and prance around together—pretending to be the mommy with small plastic babies didn't hold the charm for me it did for many of my friends. Perhaps it was no surprise that I spent a good chunk of my girlhood as a serious dance student, but during the childhood game "what do you want to be when you grow up," I never picked being a mom.

As I passed through my teens in the late sixties and early seventies, motherhood was still hardly part of the vision I held for my life in the future. I had adopted the smash-the-boundaries, culture-linked values of the time that normalized life development and self-exploration over the traditional route where marriage and family come first. Maybe it would have been different with a different mother—mine greatly supported me in attending college and developing a professional life, as well as in exploring my world. (Literally so. I spent two years in my late teens/early twenties away from my family pursuing personal goals and dreams, living first across country and then out of the country.) I will forever be grateful and proud of her wholehearted "yes" to my adventuresome inclinations.

Still, in looking back, I can see that in the sweeping excitement of opportunities and life options beginning to be legitimized for women, motherhood was not at the top of the list, culturally speaking.

At the time I thought my reticence was also due in part to feeling unsure of myself, uncertain that I would be up to the task of parenting well. Although I certainly had a lot of "the mother" within me—I did my share of mothering with friends and family, as many girls and women do—obviously, it's not quite the same as seeing yourself as a mother to a child of your own. Now as a mother, I know firsthand how this most wonderful of jobs is also one of the most demanding, I believe, in what it requires of us emotionally, intellectually, and physically. Perhaps my uncertainty was actually wisdom.

Somewhere around my mid-twenties things began to change. Once in a while, I'd find myself intently watching moms and dads with their children; with more than idle curiosity I'd wonder what it would be like to have a family of my own. By my late twenties, my occasional contemplations had transformed into a passionate longing. I still remember the first time I clearly said to myself, "I want to be a mother."

I'd tear up whenever I saw a touching picture having to do with mothers or babies. I remember the flood in finding a magazine photograph of a labor-worn yet radiant mother holding her brand-new baby in her arms. And having a child began to be a central topic in conversations with close friends. At that time I was not in a relationship with a man I wanted to have children

with, and did wonder if I ever would be. I thought about beginning a "baby bank account" just in case I'd have to go it alone.

I also earned a PhD in psychology and became a licensed marriage, family, and child counselor around that time. (At least my
capacity for caring, coupled with the therapeutic approaches I
trained in, would be of use.) Through my work with clients later
in my practice specializing in pregnancy issues, as well as through
the many conversations I've had with mothers in their middle
years in preparation for this book, I've seen how individual the
journey to motherhood can be for each of us. Yet, like me, very
often each woman clearly remembers a time of being absolutely
gripped by the feeling of wanting a baby.

I met my husband when I was 33; we were married when I
was 38. We waited a little while to settle into the state of being
married before trying to have children. It wasn't hard to wait at
that point, even though earlier I had worried about, to put it
simply, having "old eggs." I'd been anxious about the greater
chance with age of having a baby with Down syndrome as well
as about just being *able* to get pregnant in the first place as an
older woman. I knew of many women who'd had children around
their mid-thirties, but not many so close to forty. (I didn't know
at that time that *most* women even in their early forties *can* conceive and have a baby.)

My worries were for naught as far as the latter. When the time
came to try, just a couple months after I turned 39, I became
pregnant immediately.

It was wonderful. I was pregnant! My earlier concerns were
replaced by a bright new perspective, that conceiving was a snap
and that being older didn't affect a woman much when it came
to reproduction. Unfortunately, it didn't prove to be so easy. I
miscarried during my sixth week.

Going through the miscarriage was difficult. I wasn't even
showing, in fact I was far from it. But nevertheless, something real
to me, the baby, the family I had imagined we would be, the
feeling of already being a mother, had been lost.

The passage of time was healing, although I couldn't shake my worry that I might not conceive again because of my age. Nevertheless, when we tried again, I quickly became pregnant. I made it to seven weeks before this pregnancy too was lost.

Having a miscarriage often generates a lot of fear that something is wrong with your eggs or with your anatomy, or that some other flaw with your reproductive system exists that will create a miscarriage each time you conceive. My physician suggested I have the lost pregnancy tissue tested to help determine the cause. Named *karyotyping*, this kind of testing analyzes the tissue for chromosomal abnormalities.

It turned out to be an instance of reproductive bad luck. Two sperm had actually fertilized my single egg simultaneously, resulting in too many copies of each chromosome, a condition called *triploidy*. I was assured that it was totally unrelated to my age, it was a matter of unfortunate timing, and it was unlikely to occur again.

I found this news very heartening. While my first miscarriage may have been caused by an age-related problem with my egg (although we'll never know for sure), a flawed egg was not involved this second time. To my thinking it meant that I probably had plenty of good ones left. And while the fear of another miscarriage remained with me, clearly my age was no obstacle to being able to conceive.

I also went through a protocol of fertility tests around that time. Even though I had easily gotten pregnant twice and the second miscarriage was a fluke, because of my age I thought it was a good idea to do some extra investigation to move things along. When all the results were in, my doctor told me, in essence: You're fine, you're fertile, you just need a little more luck because of your age. Hearing her confirm what I believed underneath my anxiety and despite my disappointments thus far, was wonderful.

The next few months went by without my becoming pregnant. Now I was 40, and that time was something of an emotional roller coaster ride, with peaks and valleys that fluctuated many times even in a single day. Passing into my *fifth* decade of life (!) did feel like a chronological landmark, it did seem as though I had passed through a crossroads in many ways, the kind you experience when you are definitely older. While I was hardly *biologically* older since all the good-news testing, when I didn't get pregnant right away my fear that time would run out for me was intense.

At other times, however, the notion of needing "just a little luck" was calming. When I held that thought consciously, I felt optimistic. It seemed probable that at some point there *would* be that perfect egg and those perfect conditions needed for a viable pregnancy—it was just a matter of time. So it went; up when *chance* seemed like a good deal, down when concerns it wouldn't happen in time loomed large.

Then one day I had the feeling that I *would* conceive soon. The feeling was so strong that I scheduled a vacation to visit a close friend I'd been putting off. My sense was that *now* would be my last chance before my life would change by having a baby, and solo visits would be out for a while. The first month after I returned from that vacation, I became pregnant.

Did I worry about losing my pregnancy with a miscarriage? You bet. At six weeks I spotted. But the exam done at my doctor's office revealed no problems at all, and the sonogram showed a tiny, vigorously beating heart. At twenty weeks I spotted again. I was so far along, this time I had to go to the department of labor and delivery at the hospital. It was a little frightening to be there and to be surrounded by so many pieces of diagnostic medical equipment. But then too, my baby's heart was beating strong. At thirty-eight weeks, my healthy baby boy was born. Finally, I was a mother.

Overall, my pregnancy story ranks around the middle in difficulty. You may be surprised to know that the range of pregnancy experience is broad even among women with no significant reproductive problems. And age is not necessarily the best standard by which to judge who will have a textbook pregnancy and who will

face obstacles. I've spoken with women over 40 who had excep-
tional pregnancies—quick conceptions, no problems whatsoever
throughout gestation, relatively easy labors, and healthy babies.
On the other side of the age continuum, I know several women
who had one or two miscarriages during the prime of their
childbearing years, in their early and mid-twenties.

Pregnancy loss is part of the whole when it comes to having
babies. In fact, when all ages are taken together, they occur 20
percent of the time. Especially amid the initial excitement of discovering you're pregnant, this is a hard fact to consider. But if we
could, it might at least take the edge off the feeling that a violation
of the natural flow of life has occurred. This applies even more
for us in our middle years. While the facts show that *most* of us
will have successful pregnancies, our chances of experiencing a
miscarriage are greater with pregnancy later in life.

Now a midlife woman with a child, I'm a long way from my
own childhood. I find, though, that I'm still "in-between." How
so, for myself and perhaps for all of us who become mothers
during these middle years? In a potpourri of ways.

For instance, at midlife most of us are exactly that—about in
the middle of our span of years. We're not kids anymore, but not
yet seniors. We may feel youthful and look and carry ourselves
as such, and at the same time, the lines don't smooth out completely when our faces are relaxed, and we have at least glints of
gray in our hair. While many of us are quite physically active, the
days of springing up off the floor have been replaced by a graceful
but nevertheless careful climb all the way up to standing.

We are also in-between as parents, maybe beginning (or continuing) to care for our own aging mothers or fathers, at the same
time as our own infants or toddlers. We may not necessarily feel
we have a lot in common with younger mothers who grew up in
different times, but as the mothers of young children, we share
many of the same experiences and feelings. And at times the benefit of our years gives us a deeply wise, emotional knowing in

our relationships with our children, yet we can feel as helpless, overwhelmed, and impatient as a mother of any age.

Maybe being in-between as a child set the stage for pregnancy and motherhood during my middle years. It was a good fit then, as it is now. I'm thrilled that you too are looking to become pregnant and have a baby in your middle years.

Acknowledgments

My thanks to the following people:

Samuel Wood, MD, PhD, for so generously making his considerable professional expertise available to me and for reviewing *all* of the medical facts contained in this book for accuracy. My special thanks to him for all of his help.

To the midlife women I've worked with as clients dealing with pregnancy issues, and the women in their middle years who agreed to be interviewed in preparation for this book: I much appreciated being let in on your experiences with pregnancy and motherhood. Many, many thanks for sharing your stories with me.

Barbara Dixson, RN, MN, CGC (Certified Genetics Counselor); Paula Weber, RN, BSN, genetics nurse; and Gloria Anne Sanchez-Araiza, MS, MPH, CGC. For their critical review of the entire chapter on prenatal testing, the many useful sources of information they sent my way, as well as the numerous phone consultations, I am indeed most grateful.

Janice Baker, Registered Dietician, CDE (Certified Diabetes Educator) for a myriad of consultations on diet and for completely reviewing the diet and related material. All graciously done and all sincerely appreciated.

Each of the physicians I interviewed was generous with their knowledge and their time. My thanks to Carol Harter, MD; William Hummel, MD; Larry Cousins, MD; William Koltun, MD; Rosalyn Baxter-Jones, MD; Philip Milgrim, MD; as well as Kat Dalton, Certified Nurse Midwife, for her consultation.

Sincere thanks to these two physicians: Howard Schneider, MD, Director of the Neonatal Intensive Care Unit at Kaiser Permanante, San Diego Medical Center, whose consultations regarding fetal viability and review of much of that material were invaluable; and Richard Olney, MD, MPH, at the Center for Disease Control and Prevention, who spoke with me at length about folic acid and pregnancy and provided me with up-to-date, accurate information on that topic.

The California Teratogen Information Service and Clinical Research Program at the University of California San Diego Medical Center were most helpful in my efforts to gather accurate and current information on teratogens. Thanks also to Glenda Spivey, MS, President (1995–97) of OTIS, the Organization of Teratogen Information Services; and Lynn Martinez, Program Manager, Pregnancy Risk Line, Utah State Department of Health, and past President of OTIS, for their help in making referral numbers available to readers.

Acknowledgments are due to Linda Foley, MS; Marie Roberson, PhD; Margaret Thomson, RN; Robert Currier, PhD; and Sara Goldman, MPH, of the Genetic Disease Branch of California's Department of Health Services, for many discussions about the state-approved prenatal diagnosis center guidelines as well as other information related to prenatal testing; the American College of Obstetricians and Gynecologists for numerous resources on pregnancy, and especially to Greg Phillips of ACOG for making several of them available to me; Deborah Wiseman, LVN, for dialogue on an assortment of pregnancy questions; Mayland Arrington, CLS (Clinical Laboratory Scientist), owner of Claydelle Clinical Laboratory, for valuable consultations regarding pregnancy tests; and Larry Smarr, President of the Physician Insurers Association of America. My thanks also to the biomedical library staff at the University of California, San Diego, and the library staff at the North Park Library, as well to those not mentioned by name but who nevertheless also contributed to the creation of this book.

There were a number of people whose help was meaningful at a personal level. My phone conversations with Barbara Roth helped to keep my literary fires lit during the year when this book was written. She also reviewed the bulk of the manuscript and offered valuable critiques. I am grateful for all her support. The idea of writing a book came through my friendship with Rebecca Cutter, and I appreciate the support I received from her in a number of ways from early on. And I am indebted to Rick Johnson for my computer literacy on many fronts; among them, Rick taught me how to use a computer from scratch and has graciously been on call throughout to answer my emergency questions.

My thanks to Jeannette and James Trent, owners of Printcraft, for going out of their way when I needed to make copies or send faxes all those times my son was with me. Raphael Rojas helped me procure the research I needed many times when I was unable to do so myself, saving me from having to sit on my hands when there was work to be done.

Special acknowledgments to the women who took care of my son while I was writing. My thanks to Carrie Vickery and Melissa Tanbakuchi, and especially to Mary George for her gentle care and her understated kindness, and Nikia Harmon, wise about children beyond her years and there for the long haul; it was a comfort to know that my son was happy and safe during the time I worked on this book.

Last, a heartfelt thank you to my literary agent, Amy Kossow, of the Linda Allen Literary Agency, for believing in my idea for a book at the beginning, and for representing me so ably. My thanks as well to Linda Allen for her help and for being so patient with my questions when Amy was out of town. It was also my luck to work with two wonderful editors at Avon Books. Sincere thanks to Lisa Considine, my first editor, for seeing the value in the subject of midlife pregnancy and for her clear sight and perceptive eye in shaping this book into a more useful and readable form; and many thanks to Ann McKay Thoroman, my second editor at Avon, for her sure touch in fine-tuning the manuscript into a complete book.

Introduction

Why become a mother after 35? The answer to that question is easy: for the absolute, utter joy that comes with having a wanted baby; for the chance to fully mother and love unconditionally; for the enormous satisfaction in caring for one's own child and in being well used; for the fulfillment of creating a family. Beyond the tenderness and warmth, there is the pleasure in watching a young being grow, and the gratifying sense of continuity in nurturing the next generation.

For more than a few us now in our middle thirties and early forties, becoming a mother is the only piece of the pie really missing in lives that are already full and rich. Some middle-years women planned it that way, from the start not envisioning themselves as mothers until their thirties. Others wish they'd been able to have a baby earlier and have carried around an urgent, unrealized longing for many years. For still others, the strong desire for a baby is a recent, sometimes even sudden development, dawning on them from out of the blue, say, for instance, on the morning of their 39th birthday.

Regardless of where you find yourself on this continuum, midlife is a good time to have a baby. In fact, for a good number of us in our mid-thirties and beyond, now is the *right* time, even the *best* time to become a mother.

Many of us find our lives in full bloom around 35. It's an age at which many women are settled in a stable relationship, happy with their work, and perhaps financially comfortable and more relaxed with who they are than ever before. Beyond that, our chances for getting pregnant and carrying to term are generally good in our middle thirties.

It *is* wise to consider that our fertile years are not open-ended. In fact, the first appreciable reproductive changes begin around age 35, give or take a few years. Yet during the mid-thirties, while you may not have the luxury of all the time in the world to get pregnant, time is still on your side. In the chapters to come we will discuss how your blessing of time might affect your experience with pregnancy.

If you are in your forties, especially your early forties, this book offers you hope and support. What is the reality of getting pregnant at 40 and older? The reality is that although 40-plus is not a biologically optimal time to approach childbearing, for most women in their early forties, it is possible. In fact, there are more births to 40-plus women now than there have been for over 20 years.[1]

It's important to know that our reproductive systems usually undergo changes that can be dramatic around age 40. While many, many of us conceive and maintain our pregnancies with the same degree of success as younger women, it can be helpful to reshape your expectations and prepare emotionally for the 40-plus woman's journey to motherhood. In the pages ahead we will discuss why this is so as well as what you can do to best take advantage of your fertility as it is now to increase your chances of becoming pregnant.

Most women have healthy pregnancies in their midlife years. In fact, numerous medical studies have concluded there is little added risk for a midlife woman who begins her pregnancy in good health. Despite all the reassuring evidence, however, worrisome myths about having a baby at 35-plus, persist.

These myths include, for example, the beliefs that pregnancy is physically perilous for "older" women, that our bodies are not up to the task of giving birth safely, and that our chances of having an abnormal baby are great, beginning at 35. All these notions are false.

Yet even the terms often used to describe middle-years pregnancy are judgment-laden and convey nothing of the positive experience typical for older expectant mothers. Here is a sampling: "late-timed birth," "delayed childbearing," "advanced maternal age," and the particularly insulting and arcane "elderly primigravida." Although it is true that most babies are born to mothers in their twenties, 435,110 American women between the ages of 35 and 44 had babies in 1994—an average of nearly 1,200 midlife babies born every day.[2]

You may be more than taken aback to be considered a "midlife" woman. Seeing the word *midlife* applied to yourself for the first time is a little like being addressed as "ma'am" by polite children and sales clerks. You might glance around for the "mature" woman they seem to be speaking to; you're mildly shocked when you realize they're actually addressing you. Who me? I'm no "ma'am." I'm too young to be called "ma'am"! But the life expectancy for women is 79 years,[3] making 39.5 the halfway point; meaning that around 35, we open up the door to the span of time comprising our midlife years.

If you are in your mid-thirties or early forties and are thinking about having a baby, you are not alone. If you are hoping to become pregnant, or are now pregnant, you may be having a child later in life than other women, but no one can say it's too late for you to become a mother. You may have taken your time to have a baby—until it was the right time for you. The journey you're on is both common and safe; yours is, simply, a midlife pregnancy.

My criteria for choosing the material included in this book were twofold. First, that it be truly useful. I've tried to target those questions and concerns that are particularly relevant to pregnancy at midlife, as well as to cover those that are common for women of any age in the process of having a baby. Part One discusses the midlife pregnancy issues, and Part Two, the universal ones.

My second standard was that the information be up-to-date and sound. Because medicine is not only a science but also a subjective art, chances are you'll probably find differences of opinion regarding at least some of the material in these pages in any given group of physicians. Thus my job, as I saw it, was to sift through and cull out the "bottom line" from numerous and varied sources, including medical journals, consultations with medical professionals, conversations with women about their pregnancies, and my own experience.

When I was trying to conceive and when I was pregnant, I could not find the pregnancy book written for me, a *midlife* pregnant woman. There was no up-to-date, singular source that spoke to the distinct experiences and issues of women in their middle years with sufficient detail to be greatly trustworthy or useful. I have written this book to fill that gap, and I hope you will find it to be trustworthy, useful, and reassuring throughout your pregnancy.

This book is written for a woman 35 and over who is pregnant now, is hoping to become pregnant, or has just begun to think about becoming pregnant. It is also a resource for women younger than 35, wondering how possible and safe pregnancy can be in their middle years. This is a book for women of any age wanting to know about midlife pregnancy.

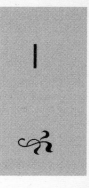

I

ABOUT PREGNANCY
LATER IN LIFE

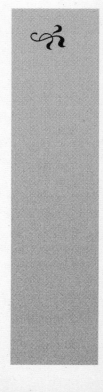

ONE

Before You Conceive

Preparing for pregnancy before conceiving is one of the smartest and most comforting steps a woman can take. Pregnancy is a thoroughly natural process, but especially when time is a point of consideration, as it is at midlife—although much less one at 35 than at 40—having all the important pieces in place means you are more likely to proceed as quickly as possible toward having a baby. This sort of efficiency is valuable, sometimes even critical, whether you are facing the limits of your fertility or whether that end point is just on the horizon.

The Time Issue

Why is time an issue—in fact *the* issue to contend with—in middle-years pregnancy? Because getting and staying pregnant *primarily* has to do with *egg quality*, and the quality of the eggs in our ovaries declines as we get older.[1]

Even when a woman hardly looks her age at 35 or 40 years old, and even when she has a good diet and may be more physically fit than ever before in her life, her healthy lifestyle and overall good condition do not change the inevitable—that is, the aging of her eggs. Unfortunately this process is both inevitable and irrevocable, as there is no way to turn back time for older eggs or to improve their basic quality.

This can be a stunning revelation for a woman who feels young and alive in every way. However, it also is not the end of the story. Despite this reproductive reality, *most midlife women, including those in their early forties, can have a baby.*[2]

Let's take a step back and work our way up to this good news. While there are some lingering questions about the when and even the whys of the decline in egg viability, it is generally accepted that fertility typically takes a distinctive dip around 35—a shift that many physicians actually don't worry much about—and then again around 39—this being the critical one in the view of many physicians.[3]

Some studies have found that first drop in a woman's fertility actually happens a little later; one pointing to the span of time between 36 and 37, another more precisely at age 37, and in a third study, 37.5 years was found to be the age when marked change was first noted.[4] What this means is that somewhere around midlife, a woman becomes "subfertile," meaning she is less fertile than younger women. This shift is not much in doubt— *it also is not necessarily a problem.* The big issue is not the fact that fertility declines as we get older. Rather, the $64,000 question is: "How does becoming subfertile actually affect a woman's chances of conceiving"?

The answer? Subfertility *does not* mean a woman has no chance of having a baby after 35; it means simply that her chances are less. In other words, although it is terribly important not to downplay the declining quality of our eggs, especially when it comes to pregnancy after 40, a woman's fertility at midlife is a relative issue and needs to be viewed in context with the whole range of fertility.

The fertility of a typical midlife woman is not unlike the singer whose voice is not what it once was, but who can hit all the right notes and still transport an audience; it's not unlike the skill of a dancer past her prime who can nevertheless still dance beautifully. Similarly, older eggs simply don't "work as well".[5] They are less able to implant in your uterus as embryos and to divide just the way needed to create a viable fetus.[6] Yet the fact is that every single day nearly 1,200 babies are born to American mothers between 35 and 44 (more than 170 of those to women in their forties).[7] Obviously, many of these eggs work just fine.

Preconception Preparations

Chances are that many of the midlife mothers who give birth to healthy babies every day were able to identify their most fertile period during the month. In fact, using ovulation predictor test kits, and learning to recognize the fertility signals present just *prior* to ovulation are the first steps in your prepregnancy preparations. Your best start on the road to a successful pregnancy includes: (1) fertility awareness (identifying ovulation and recognizing your fertility signals); (2) a basic medical exam; (3) an exam of your reproductive health; (4) genetic testing, if needed; (5) educating yourself about diet for pregnancy; and (6) gathering information about lifestyle and environmental issues that may affect your baby. Preconception care does not replace *prenatal care,* which is received during rather than before pregnancy.

Being evaluated and informed in these ways can prevent unnecessary delays in conception. For example, if you've just been immunized against German measles you'll have to wait at least three months before attempting to conceive or risk infecting and seriously damaging your baby in utero.[8] Also, educating yourself might actually decrease the time it takes to conceive because you'll have a very clear idea of when you are most fertile.

In fact, some of the newest information on successful conception is something of a departure from common beliefs about when you're likely to get pregnant, and when you're not. While you may be able to conceive as early as five days *before* you ovulate, some professionals no longer think conception is likely the day *after* ovulation.[9] Targeting those days, in addition to using ovulation predictor kits to identify the day of ovulation itself, will increase your chances each month. (Further details to follow in the section titled "Fertility Awareness".)

Second, prepregnancy education and evaluation are also beneficial because the earliest weeks of a pregnancy are critical in the growth of the tiny embryo.[10] Although many women trying to conceive are alert for signs of pregnancy, none may be apparent at the very beginning, or those that are may be confused with a pending period. By the time you have missed a period and realized you are pregnant, some of the embryo's most vital development will have already begun; under way without the benefit of knowledge leading you to take extra good care of yourself as a newly pregnant woman nourishing a newly conceived baby.

Third, any existing health problems that may affect your pregnancy (and vice versa, a medical condition you may have that could be aggravated by pregnancy) can best be dealt with now, before the fact. And the likelihood of having to make an agonizing decision, perhaps if the baby has a terminal disorder such as Tay-Sachs, is minimized by preconception testing for genetic disorders as well.

The issue here is one of *optimizing*. Although there is no guarantee with even the most thorough preparations, preconception care gives you the best shot at it by laying the foundation for a successful pregnancy. There is also a psychological benefit to knowing you've done all you could to give your baby a healthy and safe start. The vast, vast majority of babies are perfectly healthy at birth, yet most pregnant women worry about the chances of some innate problem. During those times, it can be helpful to know you've done all you could to ensure your baby's health.

Nature and Pregnancy

REPRODUCTION AND HEALTHY BABIES

Before we go further into preconception education and evaluation, a few words about nature and pregnancy. Nature, or, put another way, our biology, supports both reproduction and healthy babies. Although prepregnancy preparations can be beneficial, many, many pregnancies begin, proceed, and end very well without them, including pregnancies of women 35-plus. This is evidenced by the fact that most women who want babies not only *can* have them[11] but do so without any preliminary medical attention. Also, contrary to popular perception, the rate of birth defects is quite low, both in babies born to women of all ages, and in those with mothers over 35 as well as over 40.

As far as we know, most birth defects—not to be confused with problems such as those resulting from low birth weight, a condition that can be caused by maternal behavior—cannot be prevented by *any* level of care, either preconception or prenatal. One notable exception, neural tube defects, is believed to be minimized by early supplementing with *folic acid*. (More to follow on this.)

Birth defects generally occur in only 4 percent of all new babies.[12] They are believed to be due to problems with the egg or sperm, to a gene carried by the egg or sperm, or to some hitch in the intrinsic development of the embryo, none of which can be changed, regardless of any special attention given to the expectant mother's diet or physical health. In this country most of us don't live in places with pathologically concentrated levels of toxins. Also most Americans do get the nutrients they need even with marginal diets (fast food, junk food, sweets) although high-fat diets low in the nutrients found in fresh fruits and vegetables do create health problems such as heart disease, cancer, and obesity.[13]

THE MYTHS ABOUT STRESS

By and large, conception is ruled by biology. It seems obvious, but some of the popular beliefs that kick in—oddly enough, only when a woman *isn't* getting pregnant—have a subtext that dismisses the role biology plays in pregnancy. The problem is erroneously targeted either as a tension-related one, with advice such as: "You just need to relax," or as a psychosomatic one: "Maybe you really don't want a baby at a deep, unconscious level."

Are there connections between the body and your state of mind? Are the things you think and feel, whether conscious or unconscious, reflected in your body in various ways, such as gestures and posture? Yes. Are there instances when a woman conceives *just after* she resolves some ambivalent feelings about having a baby? Yes. Should we acknowledge an element of mystery in the timing of that woman's pregnancy? Of course.

But resolving conflicting feelings is not a prescription for getting pregnant. In fact, many of us feel some or even great ambivalence not only before, but at different times throughout pregnancy. Be very careful *not* to accept the counsel of others when they simplify and judge your situation by saying things like: "You're having trouble getting pregnant because you're not *really* ready to stop being a kid yourself."

Just as off the mark are statements like: "You're too stressed with work," or, worse, "You're too obsessed with having a baby, that's why you're not getting pregnant." Please! Unless your level of tension is so high that you are no longer menstruating and ovulating normally, stress is not the obstacle it's made out to be when it comes to conceiving. Women get pregnant during terrible, stressful times (during war and as a result of rape, for instance).

Messages like these inspire self-blame, helplessness, and anger. The circular self-talk goes something like this: I'm not getting pregnant because I'm too keyed-up, but I can't relax because I want this to happen so much. I'm worried I won't get pregnant, and that makes me even more anxious. What a Catch-22! If you are caught in this sort of vicious cycle, *stop* and consider this: No emotional state of being or psychological mindset will make you more or less likely to get pregnant. Remember that when it comes to having a baby, biology is on your side. This is as true for the woman of 42 as it is for the woman of 25. In fact, your reproductive system will not stop setting the stage for pregnancy until you literally run out of eggs or reproductive hormones.

But, because at midlife your time to have a baby is not stretching endlessly forward the way it seemed to be at 25, it makes good sense to do whatever you can to encourage a quick conception, an easy pregnancy, and a healthy baby. This ready-set-go stage also means you are making your wish for a baby more real, and perhaps more central than it was. Whether you are ready to get pregnant now or you view preconception preparations as part of the process of making a decision, these are concrete steps you can take toward motherhood. Now on to the details of preconception care, beginning with fertility awareness.

Fertility Awareness

OVULATION PREDICTION TEST KITS

The best way to determine when you're ovulating is with an ovulation prediction kit. These at-home urine tests measure levels of luteinizing hormone, or LH, in your system. This reproductive hormone is directly responsible for the release of an egg from one of your ovaries.[14] Color changes in a test vial indicate when the amount of luteinizing hormone surges, which occurs right before ovulation.[15] You will probably ovulate at some point within those next twenty-four hours.

According to some of the newer thinking about timing conception, your chances of conceiving are much greater *up to and through* the day of ovulation, than after.[16] Thus, the twenty-four hours after you detect the surge of LH signaling ovulation are thought to be the time conception is *most* likely.[17]

One note of caution here for midlife women, especially those over 40: If your test indicates an LH surge—that is, it changes from a light to an unmistakably intense shade of blue—and the test results remain the same for more than two days, you may not be detecting ovulation but rather early menopause, a time also associated with high levels of LH.[18] Speak to your physician if this happens to you. You will quite possibly undergo some lab tests to determine if you are unexpectedly menopausal or be referred for further evaluation by a fertility specialist.

FERTILITY SIGNALS

Becoming aware of your own fertility signals improves your chances of having a baby. While you are *most* fertile on the day you ovulate, a recent study has suggested that *several* days just before ovulation are also important. Pregnancy is thought to be a possibility when you have intercourse up to five keys before an egg is released. This gives a woman a "fertile" period totaling six days (the five days before, plus the day of ovulation itself).[19]

This relatively broad six-day "window of conception" is a function of the potential longevity of your partner's sperm and the receptivity of the cervical mucus.[20] Although these days do not all offer *equal* chances—the two days before and especially the day of ovulation being far and away the best times[21]—to take advantage of all these favorable days, you must learn to read when you are *approaching* ovulation—when you are in that window.

Reading the signs of pending ovulation will not make it possible to pinpoint when the first of those days begin before the fact. But these signs will give you clues that can help you make an educated guess about whether you are within that six-day period.

Here are the nuts and bolts involved in reading your fertility signals: You are looking for: (1) changes in cervical fluid or mucus (your most reliable clue in identifying your fertile period); (2)

changes in the cervix itself; and (3) "mittelschmerz" or lower abdominal pain associated with ovulation.

CERVICAL MUCUS

Your cervical mucus usually becomes clear, semiliquid, slip-
pery, and stretchy in consistency as ovulation nears; this mucus
is thought to nourish and protect sperm before and through ovulation. Chances are, by the time you notice it, you will be fast approaching if not already within the six-day window, depending
on the progress of your own individual cycle.

Watch for changes in cervical mucus when you are using the
toilet or changing your underwear. It may become even more fluid
and more voluminous on the day of ovulation itself, although the
peak mucus day for some women may actually occur one or two
days before or after ovulation.[22]

Some factors can affect the appearance of your cervical fluids,
and therefore your ability to recognize whether you are clearly in
a fertile phase. A vaginal infection can easily disguise the charac-
teristic textures described above. Yeast infections, for instance,
cause a discharge that is opaque and whitish, mimicking the fluid
present in the earlier, nonfertile part of your cycle.

Residual semen and lubricants such as K-Y Jelly can also look
very much like the clear, stretchy cervical fluid you're watching
for. So much so that you might mistake either of these semiliquid
fluids for fertile mucus and assume your fertile period has come
and gone. Some couples unintentionally cut back on having sex
regularly throughout the month during the period of time they
are trying to have a baby. As their focus shifts from having sex
together to baby-making, they end up strategically planning intercourse *only* for those days they believe conception is possible. If
this is so for you, simply be sure to check your cervical mucus
each day. That way, you won't miss your fertile days or any opportunities for getting pregnant that month. Also, be sure to check

with your physician about using a lubricant, as some believe they can impede sperm making their way to fertilize an egg.[23]

Birth control pill usage can also cause some confusion about your pre-ovulation phase. The *combination* birth control pills most commonly used essentially work by preventing the production of hormones related to ovulation, thereby suspending the process of maturation and release of an egg.[24] When you stop taking the Pill in order to get pregnant, it may take a while for the production of reproductive hormones, ovulation, and menstruation to normalize.[25] In fact, you may temporarily stop menstruating altogether. However, unless you have (without realizing it) moved close or into early menopause while on the Pill, you will become fertile again. Meanwhile, you will want to pay close attention to your fertility signals on a daily basis.

Cycle patterns and the changes in your cycle as you age are quite individual. More or less subtle alterations you may have noticed as you moved into your late twenties and early thirties, usually become pronounced by your late thirties. For instance, women who once could count the precise number of days between periods may now have some shorter or longer cycles. The woman who always had a range of days she could count on (most of us) may notice that the duration of menstruation is shorter, the flow of cervical fluid seems diminished, or the number of days per cycle are usually fewer, or, more commonly, greater than before.

If you feel you need help in recognizing your fertile mucus, speak with your doctor. Be sure to consult your doctor if no such mucus is at all apparent.

MITTELSCHMERZ

The release of an egg from the ovary causes some women a degree of pain ranging from a mild twinge to a severe ache, anywhere from the side to the center of their lower abdomen. This is often referred to by the Yiddish term *mittelschmerz*,[26] meaning "middle pain."[27] Although it can be uncomfortable, the woman who experiences mittelschmerz is most fortunate, as this is a definite sign of ovulation, her most fertile time.

Look for this twinge/ache around the middle of your cycle during a phase of fertile mucus. Sometimes sitting down off-balance or hard can trigger the sensation of pain from ovulation. It is possible that by simply fine-tuning your awareness you will detect the presence of this body signal. If you simply don't experience mittelschmerz, there are a few other signs to look for in addition to fertile cervical mucus.

First, some women experience a heightened interest in being sexual around the time of ovulation. Said a friend of mine, "I know I'm about to ovulate when I want to make love much more than usual, and the desire lasts for two or three days in a row. It happens every month around the middle of my cycle, even when I've been busy all day and feel tired by the time we go to bed." If you experience this sort of "psychobiological" arousal, count yourself lucky and use this awareness to your advantage. Other women may not notice any such urge, but rather simply have an intuitive sense that they will get pregnant if they have intercourse at a particular time. If you have such a feeling, act on it.

CERVICAL CHANGES

One other physical sign may help you identify your fertile phase, in the form of your cervix itself. You may notice that your cervix will change in its firmness as you move close to ovulation.

While not every woman will notice these changes, the fertile cervix often feels substantive but relatively soft to the touch, with some give to it as if you were to gently press on the tip of your nose. When you are not fertile, your cervix will generally be firm to the touch. This cue can help you confirm the judgment you've already made that the time of ovulation is getting close based on the appearance of your cervical mucus.

Your body signals can be a valuable adjunct to your biochemical ovulation predictor test. Timing is so critical to becoming pregnant. While the kits will help you pinpoint ovulation, these signs will give you direct and immediate feedback during the pre-ovulatory period of the month. Most midlife women, although subfertile, are nevertheless still fertile. After 35 and into the forties conceiving may not happen as easily, but most of us can conceive. And practicing fertility awareness makes your chances of having a baby even better.

Preconception Exams and Evaluations

The primary purpose of a preconception medical exam is to discover any underlying problems that could potentially flare up during pregnancy. The primary purpose of the evaluation of your general reproductive health is twofold: to detect any obvious fertility problems, and to test both your immunity against certain diseases and the existence of active infections that could affect either your pregnancy or your baby in utero.

THE PRECONCEPTION PHYSICAL

Your preconception medical exam is similar to an annual physical. Your physician (probably a family or primary care doctor) will take a history, examine you, and conduct or order tests such as blood and urine analysis to check your overall health.

Anything out of the ordinary should be dealt with before you become pregnant. Chronic high blood pressure, diabetes, anemia, and epilepsy are among the pre-existing medical conditions that might create complications during pregnancy.[28] Pregnancy concerns aside, the first two affect midlife women to a greater extent simply because they occur more often as we get older. (*Fibroids* are a third medical issue more common for women in their middle years that may then cause pregnancy-related problems. I'll talk about them in the next section on the preconception reproductive health exam.)

High blood pressure, or hypertension, is a condition in which your blood travels through your arteries with more force than is normal. The undue pressure on the walls of your arteries can lead to a host of medical problems, ranging from light-headedness to heart attacks.[29] Women with chronic high blood pressure are more likely to develop a complication known as *pregnancy-induced hypertension* or *preeclampsia* during their pregnancies. The blood supply to the placenta, through which the fetus is nourished, diminishes when a woman has this condition.[30]

(Preeclampsia may *also* develop more frequently during the pregnancies of women over 35. Thus for such women there are both an age/hypertension/preeclampsia link and an age-when-pregnant/preeclampsia link, to be aware of—though not necessarily to be overly concerned about. Later in this chapter we'll look at the commonsense approach to pregnancy risks after 35.)

When a person has *diabetes,* the body cannot maintain a normal balance of insulin and glucose on its own.[31] Miscarriage and birth defects are among the problems that occur more often when this condition is not brought under control prepregnancy.[32]

(*Gestational* diabetes can also develop after you become pregnant because of the effect of pregnancy hormones on insulin.[33] This too is a condition that may occur more often in midlife pregnancy.[34])

Discovering that you have high blood pressure or diabetes and getting treatment and advice before pregnancy are positive steps toward having a safe and healthy pregnancy. Although many medical problems that worsen or arise *during* gestation can be dealt with successfully, it is a definite advantage to get them well controlled beforehand. Beyond the benefit of any immediate medical care, your doctor will also be forewarned about the need to monitor your condition when you are pregnant.

THE PRECONCEPTION REPRODUCTIVE HEALTH EXAM

Like the preconception medical exam, this evaluation of your reproductive health is similar to your annual gynecological exam. Conducted by your obstetrician-gynecologist, its two main components are (1) a basic fertility check and (2) screening for the presence of harmful infections and immunity against certain pregnancy-adverse diseases.

Your Fertility

A basic fertility check first and foremost involves a discussion of whether you are ovulating. Initially, your doctor may be listening for your report of signs of ovulation, such as an increase in mucus or mittelschmerz (pain in your abdomen with the release of an egg).[35] He or she may check the level of the hormone *progesterone* in your blood in the second half of your cycle to confirm whether you are ovulating normally.[36] Or you may be asked to chart your *basal body temperature* (taken before rising) to look for the slight increase that shows up after ovulation.[37]

You will probably be asked questions regarding endometriosis, a condition in which the tissue that ordinarily lines the uterus grows outside of it, often in places that some medical doctors believe interferes with fertility. Typical questions are: Do you have menstrual cramps? Do you have pain with intercourse? A positive response to both may be cause for further examination.

Whether endometriosis adversely affects a woman's fertility is in question. Some physicians believe it plays a major role and others, a minimal one.[38] However, there's no doubt that it occurs more frequently in older women—the average age it appears is 37, and it is more common in women who have not had babies earlier in their lives.[39] Because a problem could mean you'll need to put off trying to get pregnant while you undergo treatment, questions about endometriosis will most likely be part of your fertility check.

You will also be examined for fibroid tumors. Exactly how and to what extent fibroids might affect a pregnancy is also a subject of controversy.[40] While they are more common for women at midlife, some professionals do not believe these benign uterine tumors cause pregnancy problems very often.[41] Nevertheless, knowing that you have fibroids before you conceive will give you time to discuss with your doctor whether you need treatment, and to consider the options available.

Last, you will be asked if your mother took DES, short for *diethylstilbestrol* to prevent miscarriage or preterm labor when she was pregnant with you. This drug was found to cause structural uterine and cervical abnormalities in "DES daughters."[42] It has also been linked with a rare vaginal or cervical cancer called *clear-cell cancer*.[43] The drug was prescribed to women between 1938 and 1971[44] but most widely used in the 1950s. Hence many DES daughters are now in their midlife years.

If you already know or believe there is a possibility that you were exposed to diethylstilbestrol in utero, be sure to work with a physician knowledgeable about the effects of DES. A DES examination differs in some slight but important ways from the exam you routinely receive from your regular ob/gyn.[45]

Even obvious structural abnormalities, however, aren't necessarily a guarantee of pregnancy difficulties. In fact, *most* DES daughters don't have special pregnancy problems.[46] Yet some problems do occur more often among this group—tubal pregnancy, preterm labor, and miscarriage have been associated with DES—so you will want to receive some extra monitoring right from the start if you are a DES daughter.[47]

Infections and Immunity

The second component of your preconception ob/gyn exam involves screening for the presence of infections and verifying your immunity to a number of diseases. Some active infections and diseases can cause birth defects. Some treatment options are safe for use during pregnancy, but others are not. For instance, women are usually advised to wait at least three months after receiving a vaccination before trying to conceive, to avoid exposing the fetus.[48] Some vaccines do not provide lifetime protection, so you may well need to receive a new immunization.[49] While many, if not most of us, will have clean results on all of these tests, when it comes to checking infections and your immunity status, the earlier you get a clean bill of health from your doctor, the better.

Your doctor should check for the following:

INFECTIONS

Chlamydia, genital herpes, gonorrhea, and syphilis

Toxoplasmosis

HIV

• *Chlamydia, genital herpes, gonorrhea, and syphilis*
These diseases are all caused by sexual contact with an infected partner.[50]

• *Toxoplasmosis*
Toxoplasmosis is caused by a parasite found in undercooked meats, raw milk, and cat feces.[51] This infection can cause serious birth defects in the fetus, affecting the brain and eyes.[52] Be careful when digging in your garden with bare hands and when cleaning the cat box. If you're trying to conceive, use gloves and wash your hands thoroughly afterward, or better yet, delegate those tasks.

• *HIV*
Presently, it is mandatory in some states that health care providers offer counseling and testing for HIV.[53] If in the future it is shown that transmission of HIV from infected mother to fetus is cut down when treatment is received during pregnancy, then the question of mandatory testing will probably be on the table. However as things stand now you can choose to be tested for HIV or not. A positive result would have enormous ramifications for you and your hoped-for child, but only you can make this decision.

If it helps you to hear yourself think out loud, turn to a trusted friend or counselor to talk about your thoughts and feelings. And as with all the medical issues outlined in this book, discuss your questions about the facts involved in HIV testing with your doctor. Physicians are required by law to maintain your confidentiality. Neither the specifics of your concerns nor the results of testing can be released without your written permission (with one exception: the unlikely possibility that your medical records are subpoenaed by a court as part of a legal proceeding). Also, testing for HIV at home is possible with the Confide HIV Test Kit manufactured by Johnson and Johnson. It is available over the counter at many pharmacies, costing around $40.

IMMUNITY[54]

Rubella (German measles)

Hepatitis B

Measles

Mumps

Polio

Tetanus-diphtheria

* *Rubella (German measles)*
Rubella is passed around by the droplets spread when a person infected with this virus coughs or sneezes. Rubella can cause severe birth defects in the baby exposed in utero during the first trimester, such as heart disorders, cataracts (which can lead to blindness), deafness, and mental retardation.[55]

Having a bout with this disease once gives you lifelong immunity.[56] If you received a vaccination as a child, however, your doctor may want to do a blood test to be sure you are still immune.[57] If a new or first vaccination is needed, you will want to be immunized early in your preconception preparations. You must wait at least three months after receiving it before trying to conceive to guard against the possibility of transmitting the virus contained in the vaccine to the fetus.[58]

- *Hepatitis B*

Hepatitis B, or HBV, is caused by a virus that affects the liver.[59] HBV can be passed to another person by blood, through kissing, or through intercourse.[60] Some infected people have no symptoms but may pass the disease on as a lifelong carrier of the virus. Most babies born to mothers with HBV become infected. These babies may go on to develop serious medical problems such as cirrhosis or hardening of the liver and usually become carriers themselves.[61]

Your doctor will advise you to become immunized if he or she believes you are at risk for contracting Hepatitis B. This vaccine is given in three doses that are administered over the course of seven months.[62]

- *Measles*

Many of us developed an immunity to measles the hard way when we contracted this viral disease as children. The positive side is the lifelong immunity the sufferer thus acquires.[63] A woman who received a vaccine as a child will want to check with her doctor just in case he or she believes a new vaccine is warranted. If you have not had the disease or have never been vaccinated against measles, you'll want to be immunized at least three months before pregnancy. You don't want to expose the fetus to the live virus used for this purpose.[64] Measles are spread by contact with little droplets from the nose, mouth, and throat of an infected person.[65]

- *Mumps*

Mumps is spread through contact with the saliva of a person infected by this virus.[66] It is rare in adults; however, your chances of a miscarriage double if you become infected in your first trimester, and mumps may also put you at higher risk for preterm labor later in pregnancy.[67] Women without immunity to mumps are not given vaccinations while they are pregnant as the vaccine poses some risk to the baby, albeit a small one. Again, medical advice is to wait at least three months after immunization before trying to conceive to protect the baby from exposure to the live virus used for the mumps vaccine.[68]

- *Polio*

Most of us in our midlife years were immunized against polio as children. However, while the polio vaccine itself does not pose a danger during pregnancy,[69] pregnant women more often get the paralytic than the mild form of this disease.[70] Although all forms of polio are rare today,[71] women who are not immune should get the vaccine before they try to conceive to ensure their own protection.

- *Tetanus-diphtheria*

You may also want to check to be sure your tetanus-diphtheria immunization is up to date. Boosters are given at ten-year intervals.[72] If you are soon due for one, your doctor may advise you to receive it prepregnancy.

SAVING ON COSTS

The exam formats outlined here are not complete but rather highlight some important features when you are preparing for pregnancy. The form preconception physicals and ob/gyn exams take will vary from physician to physician. Yours may well be more extensive depending on your doctor's standard practices and judgment based on your individual medical history.

Much of what is involved in these exams is already a part of your annual physical and ob/gyn checkups. To cut down on additional costs, consult with your doctor. Your physician may believe some of the tests could be safely eliminated based on his or her knowledge of your health and individual medical background.

Also, being thoroughly examined by both your family doctor and your ob/gyn will mean some overlap that doesn't necessarily bring you any benefit. (Each may take a family and medical history, each may check your blood pressure, etc.) To avoid paying for two office visits, you may be able to combine these two exams into one conducted by your ob/gyn.

SAVING TIME (AND ASSURING A HEALTHY START)

Prepregnancy evaluations are especially valuable to midlife women because of the time issue. If you are waiting to first have your preconception exam before trying to get pregnant, and find that you are putting off making an appointment, you may be losing valuable time, particularly if you are in your late thirties or early forties.

It's a good idea to have these exams because fertility problems or health issues that are unknown to you might cause even more of a delay in the long run. Endometriosis that forms on your ovaries might hamper ovulation itself, for example. When a problem that diminishes your chances for conceiving are diagnosed and treated *before* you start trying to get pregnant, you may be saving yourself from many wasted months as well as a great deal of worry and unnecessary frustration.

Diseases that tax your body could be much more dangerous to a fetus, so it's important, for instance, to check on your vaccination record early. You might avoid needing to take a three-month break when you're already in the process of attempting to conceive, if you later discover you're missing an important one. No expectant mother wants to be exposed to rubella or any other potentially harmful disease without having the immunity to protect her vulnerable developing baby.

However, having periods that are normal and regular, recognizing those signs that confirm you are ovulating, being in good health and certain that your immunization status is fairly complete, and knowing you have steered clear of experiences that could pose a risk to your baby in utero—such as possible exposure to the AIDS virus—are all reasons to feel positive about your fertility and your health. You may decide you are comfortable with the prospect of dealing with any possible problems that become apparent down the road, and try to become pregnant first.

PRECONCEPTION GENETIC TESTING

The occurrence of genetic disorders that are *inherited* is *not* age related, as the case is with genetic problems caused by chromosomal abnormalities, such as Down syndrome.[73] In other words, being older does not mean you are any more likely than a younger woman to be a carrier of a gene for cystic fibrosis, for example, or to pass it on to your children.

Some disorders seem to run in families; others are more common in women and men of certain ethnic groups. For example, Tay-Sachs occurs more frequently in Jewish people of East European descent (Ashkenazi Jews); thalassemia is more often found in persons of Mediterranean and Asian origins; and sickle-cell anemia is more frequent in African-Americans.[74] If a genetic disorder runs in your family, or if you are a member of one of these groups, it will be important for you to have preconception genetic testing.

Genetic testing can also detect the presence of genes for particular diseases that might be passed from parent to child. The father of the baby may also be screened to determine whether he might be a carrier.[75] Testing can also often tell you what the chances are that your baby may inherit a genetic disorder. Some disorders can be passed only if both parents are carriers, others if only one parent is.

When either or both parents are carriers, knowing the degree of probability that their child will receive the defective gene for that particular disease beforehand is an enormous benefit. Prior knowledge allows you to prepare in advance for a child with a major disease or to avoid having to deal with the difficult issue of considering an abortion when you are already pregnant.

Preconception Diet and Weight

DIET

Whether or not you are eating the recommended amounts of fruits and vegetables, grains and meats, calcium-rich foods, and fats, prepregnancy is the best time to fine-tune your diet.

As an expectant mother, you'll feel good making sure your nutrition is optimal in the first weeks and months of pregnancy when the organs, spine, and musculature of your baby are beginning to form.[76] Further, if the quality of your diet has been erratic, or you are a long-term dieting veteran without a real sense of what normal eating actually is, you can use this time to become familiar and comfortable with a basic balanced diet.

The summary below shows what makes up a complete diet.[77] You will find an expanded version in Appendix B, listing foods and exact serving sizes.

Protein foods: 2–3 servings/day

Calcium-rich foods: 2–3 servings/day

Fruits: 2–4 servings/day

Vegetables: 3–5 servings/day

Grains, breads, and cereal: 6–11 servings/day

Fluids: at least six 8-ounce glasses/day (not counting caffeinated or alcoholic beverages)

Fats: Limit to no more than 30 percent of total calorie intake

Eating a variety of foods from each group in the amounts suggested should provide all the nutrients you need to get started on a nutritionally optimal pregnancy.[78] However, you will want to pay special attention to the following nutrients.

Folate (folic acid). The use of this B vitamin has been associated with a decrease in the incidence of neural tube defects such as spina bifida and anencephaly.[79] Tomatoes, green leafy vegetables, cauliflower, bananas, and orange juice are good sources.[80] However, because of this link, a *supplement* of 400 micrograms is recommended for *all* women in their childbearing years, even those not planning on pregnancy, just in case.[81] (In addition, as of January 1998, fortification with folic acid is required by the Food and Drug Administration for flours and many flour products identified as *enriched*.[82])

It is most important to take in the recommended amounts of this vitamin before pregnancy—a good reserve of folic acid in place *beforehand* ensures that a good supply is ready and waiting for the newly conceived baby to draw upon, through at least the sixth week, dated from the first day of your last menstrual period (or your fourth week after conception), when the neural tube develops.[83] The American College of Obstetricians and Gynecologists recommends that you supplement with 400 micrograms of folate throughout your first trimester.[84]

The recommended daily amounts of folic acid are periodically updated. Check with your doctor about the most current recommendations when you discuss your preconception supplement plans with him or her.

Iron. Iron is found in meats, eggs, dried fruit, and spinach.[85] Many women do not get enough in their regular diet.[86] Although you can make up for a minimal iron intake during pregnancy—in fact, iron supplements are often prescribed as pregnancy progresses (usually in the second or third trimester)—having an adequate supply now will help you begin your pregnancy feeling strong and healthy.

However, supplementing with iron on a generic basis is no longer considered wise. A serious disease called *hemochromatosis*, involving toxic levels of iron reserves in the liver, although not widespread, has been found to be much more common than once thought. So be *very* sure to speak with your doctor before increasing your iron intake. Chances are he or she will have your blood screened for iron levels, especially if any family members have hemochromatosis.[87]

Calcium. Milk, yogurt, cheese, and broccoli are all good sources of calcium.[88] This mineral is crucial to bone and tooth development; is important to nerve, muscle, and heart development; and is needed for blood clotting, among other specialized functions.[89] Although all women need to take in enough calcium to help prevent osteoporosis from developing when older (usually not until after menopause) women planning on becoming pregnant have an extra factor to consider; the fetus will actually leech the calcium it needs from the mother's bones if she does not consume an adequate amount, making her bones susceptible to osteoporosis later. Calcium is an important nutrient overall to be aware of and include in your prepregnancy diet.

Fluids. Fluids include water and water-based liquids such as juices, and *decaffeinated* coffee and teas. (Caffeine counterproductively acts as a diuretic.[90]) Fluids move toxins through the body and hydrate your whole system. If you have not been a big water drinker, when you begin taking in adequate fluids you may find that you feel better physically.

WEIGHT

Those of us going into pregnancy overweight at midlife may be more likely to develop pregnancy-induced hypertension and maternal diabetes, as weight has been associated with these gestational problems,[91] as has age.[92] Starting out at a higher weight means you'll become that much heavier as the gestational months go by, also making you more susceptible to general pregnancy discomfort.

Yet many of us are a few pounds or so over our ideal weights and we do just fine, progressing through pregnancy without a hitch. If you have any questions about your body size and pregnancy, be sure to discuss with your doctor whether weight loss is a must, a "soft" recommendation for you, or not an issue at all. Ask about the pluses of losing weight and consequences of not.

Preconception-wise body size can be an issue at the *extremes* of thin or overweight. Some physicians contend that being too thin or very overweight can affect fertility by affecting hormone levels, causing irregular cycles or even bringing ovulation to a halt.[93] Others believe the link between body size and the production of the reproductive hormone estrogen, or to be specific, the link between percentage of *body fat* and estrogen, is rarely a sole factor causing a problem with ovulation; rather, excessive thinness or overweight more often plays a corollary role to other factors that interfere with egg production. (For instance, an eating disorder, such as anorexia, or marathon running may affect ovulation.[94] More on heavy exercising in the next section.)

If you are either very thin or overweight and not ovulating, your doctor may consider body fat percentage as at least a possible contributing factor. If you are ovulating, body size is not a fertility issue to worry about. However, if you are at either extreme there may be other concerns. For example, a very thin woman may not eat enough to supply adequate nutrition for either her baby or herself when she is pregnant. Women who are obese may have approximately two to three times the risk of having a baby with a neural tube defect—especially spina bifida—according to two recent studies.[95] Obese women may also be at higher risk for stillbirth.[96] Any health and weight issues—bulimia is another example—are best dealt with preconception.

Lifestyle and Environmental Issues

EXERCISE

Exercise can be an enormous plus to a pregnant woman. Being physically fit can help you better weather the discomforts of pregnancy, might make you more efficient in labor, and can speed up recovery after delivery. These are terrific reasons to remain active or to begin exercising prepregnancy if you are not already involved in sports or working out.

To support your pregnancy and labor experience, participate in aerobic exercise for endurance, and work your whole body for strength, concentrating on thighs, hips, and abdomen. If you have been relatively sedentary, consult your doctor for advice about the best and safest ways to build up your stamina and muscle tone.

A prepregnancy caution, however, about heavy exercising: Those women engaged in very taxing forms of exercise, such as ballet dancers and triathletes, may find a link between their extraordinary level of activity and their fertility.[97] As with body size, the guideline here is very simple. If you are involved in unusually demanding kinds of activity, and your cycles are irregular or you are not ovulating, your doctor may conclude that your level of exercise is at least a contributing factor. Your doctor may advise you to cut back and may run some tests to look further into your fertility.

ALCOHOL

The adverse effects of alcohol on a developing fetus run the gamut from the loss of a few IQ points to an obviously impaired child with the facial malformations and mental retardation that characterize fetal alcohol syndrome.[98] Alcohol interferes with brain development, that much is known. What is not known, however, is exactly how much alcohol is safe.[99]

Do not venture into motherhood if presently you are actively alcoholic. The potential harm to the fetus, and the adverse emotional and psychological consequences for children of alcoholics, make this a very clear-cut issue. Heavy drinkers must deal with their alcohol dependency before pregnancy.

The enormous physical and emotional demands that will be made on you in raising a child and especially in caring for a newborn are also reasons to quit now. Counseling with a reputable professional and group support through programs such as Alcoholics Anonymous can help you stop drinking. You must find an alternative way of dealing with difficult feelings, something self-supportive and life affirming, as you will in all probability be stretched to your limits and beyond many times as a mother. Whether or not you subscribe to the theory that alcoholism is a physiological reaction, a solid resolution will mean both zero drinking and working through the emotional issues tied into your drinking.

Many women who drink socially choose to forgo alcohol entirely during pregnancy—as well as during the time they are trying to conceive. While it takes five to seven days after conception before the embryo implants and begins receiving nutrients from the mother,[100] few women know they're pregnant this early. The embryo will of course receive any toxic substances that are also in the mother's system.

While some argue that wine is much more a regular part of life in Europe and there's no big news about babies born alcohol damaged—a comforting thought for those women who inadvertently have alcoholic beverages during the earlier stages of an unexpected pregnancy—for many, the possibility of affecting fetal development and causing harm to their baby by having drinks with dinner or at a party once they suspect they are pregnant or know for sure is not a worthwhile risk.

SMOKING

Smoking has been associated with an increase in stillbirths—the more you smoke, the higher the risk[101]—and with low birth weight babies—born almost twice as often to smoking mothers as to nonsmoking mothers.[102] Sudden infant death syndrome has also been linked to tobacco use.[103]

Obviously, some mothers-to-be do smoke, and many, many more did so throughout pregnancy in the past before smoking was stigmatized. Most of their babies turned out fine. However, why take the chance? Preconception is the best time to quit; if you can't entirely, the more you cut back and the fewer cigarettes you smoke per day, the better.

CAFFEINE AND MARGINAL FERTILITY

Caffeine may make conception less likely for women taking in more than 115 milligrams per day.[104] A single 6-ounce cup of ground coffee will have from 80 milligrams up to 200 milligrams if the brew is very strong; a 6-ounce cup of percolated coffee, from 110 to 160 milligrams. Six ounces of instant coffee contains 55 to 85 milligrams and there are 25–70 milligrams of caffeine in the same amount of tea.[105] However, although it is important to realize that caffeine is actually a drug, it's possible that the negative effects matter only when a woman's fertility is already marginal. Then an additional adverse element, like too much caffeine, might push the possibility of conceiving just over the line.

Yet unless there is an obvious sign of a problem, such as irregular periods, or until sufficient time has passed and you've proven to be infertile, how do you know you're at the margins?

The most cautious approach is to simply eliminate or to limit your total caffeine intake to 115 milligrams per day. (Chocolate lovers: Caffeine is contained in chocolate, however, 115 milligrams would require eating a considerable amount, from about 12 to 23 ounces depending on the caffeine content.[106]) If your morning coffee or tea is important to you, speak with your doctor. If he or she doesn't see a problem, caffeine intake will be one less preconception concern.

PRESCRIPTION DRUGS

Medications prescribed by your doctor are not necessarily safe for use when you are pregnant. For example, Accutane, an oral acne medication, not only can cause serious birth defects, but remains potent in your system even after you stop taking it. A woman using it will probably be advised to stop, then wait *at least* one month before trying to conceive, to be sure it's been completely eliminated from her body.[107]

Some *psychotropic* drugs—the class of medications taken for conditions such as depression, anxiety, or schizophrenia, for example—may be teratogenic (cause birth defects). Although only a few are thought to increase the risk of birth defects, and even then only slightly,[108] you should consult the prescribing physician about the effects on the fetus of any medication you are taking.

Give yourself as much time as possible before conception to make the transition if alternative medication is necessary. Sometimes it takes a while before the right dosages or mixtures of psychotropics are found. Or, if you decide to discontinue your medication while you are pregnant, doing so gradually may be critical.

Conversely, the system-wide changes your body goes through in pregnancy may alter the effectiveness of your preconception dosage. It may need to be adjusted once you are pregnant to adequately meet your treatment needs.[109]

ENVIRONMENTAL CHEMICALS

There are thousands of toxins in our environment.[110] At home, at work, and outdoors you are likely to encounter some. There is no way to identify and test each one, either those that are man-made or those that are natural. Here are some basic guidelines to help you monitor your preconception exposure to environmental chemicals, along with a list of substances known to be potentially harmful during pregnancy.

First, are you required to wear a mask or apron on the job? Such gear may be a precaution to protect you from toxic exposure that might well cause birth defects.[111] If you use any sort of protective clothing or gear at work, investigate to identify the toxic source. Then learn all you can about the potential harm to your baby.

Speak with your doctor or a genetics counselor for information. You might also wish to contact a *teratogen information service*—a program that offers women telephone consultations to answer specific questions about teratogens. Your doctor or a genetics counselor may be able to give you the phone number of such a service in your region or state. Not all states have these programs in place, and many are only able to handle calls from residents. However, you can call the following numbers for referral information: If you live east of the Mississippi River, call the Pregnancy/Environmental Hotline in Massachusetts, at (617) 466–8474; west of the Mississippi, try the Pregnancy Risk Line at (801) 328–2229, located in Utah.[112]

While your exposure to teratogens does not, fortunately, mean birth defects are inevitable, you will want to take precautions. *Now* is the time to make a plan if necessary to eliminate or reduce your exposure while you're pregnant, such as by requesting a transfer to another work area that is safe for your baby. Protection against known or potential teratogens in your environment is especially important during the first trimester when the developing embryo is most vulnerable. Far better to be inconvenienced or pushy than risk a birth defect.

Next, if your contact with a chemical makes you sick, it more than likely will make your developing baby sick too. So if you were poisoned by drinking a toxic chemical or breathing in dangerous fumes, your baby is probably also at risk. However, if you inhale a spray that has a disgusting smell, in fact smells so bad you can't imagine it is not hazardous to the health of human beings, but you don't become nauseated (not counting the sensitivity that is part of morning sickness) or weak, or faint, probably your baby is entirely unaffected.[113]

Here is a list of known teratogens, which you should avoid during pregnancy: lead, mercury, ceramics and pottery glaze containing lead, and the chemicals involved in the process of making paint, glass, or batteries.[114] While the chemicals in dry cleaning solutions and in the acrylic used in manicuring acrylic nails have not been proven to be teratogenic, some physicians also advise their patients to avoid these substances as a precaution.[115] Be sure to let your doctor know if you work with or around any of these materials.

You may feel better ventilating well and wearing gloves as a precaution when using cleaning products while cleaning the kitchen or bathroom with them. Stay entirely away if walls with any layers of old paint are being scraped or torn down, to avoid breathing in lead. Wait at least until the paint dust is neither floating nor anywhere present.

Prepregnancy is also the time to check your water supply for lead content as well as overall safety and purity. Call your local public utilities if you use tap water, or the distributor of your bottled water company for their latest test results; they should check for impurities regularly. Doing so before you conceive will give you time to investigate to your satisfaction and let you be comfortable with your water source.

Pregnancy Risks at Midlife: The Myths and Realities

MIDLIFE PREGNANCY—SAFE PREGNANCY

The long-held, entrenched belief that having a baby is chock-full of risks for an older woman is by and large an outdated one. The best evidence of this shift is that healthy 35-plus pregnant women are routinely cared for by their regular ob/gyns rather than by physicians who specialize in following high-risk pregnancies (*perinatologists*). This level of comfort is probably based on a great deal of positive experience with older pregnant patients; in other words, the actual, factual pregnancy experience of midlife women themselves has probably done the most to change minds.

This is a powerful statement about the general safety of late-in-life pregnancy, considering the financial risks involved in practicing medicine. Relatively few physicians will consciously expose themselves to a malpractice suit by providing care for a patient whose needs are beyond their expertise. This is probably especially true in obstetrics. Obstetricians/gynecologists rank either first or in the top three in every state in the frequency of medical claims brought against them and in the dollar amount of malpractice insurance they must carry.[116]

MIDDLE YEARS MOTHERS PAST AND PRESENT

Having a baby in your mid-thirties and forties is hardly anything new. For instance, in the mid-1920s, the average age for having a last baby was 42.[117] Around 50 years ago, the percentage of midlife women having babies was nearly double and triple the number of women in the same age range that are having children today.[118] In 1945, approximately 57 in 1,000 women aged 35 to 39 gave birth, as compared to about 34 in 1,000 in 1994. And back then, around 17 in 1,000 women in their early forties had babies, with just over 6 in 1,000 doing so in 1994.

(These statistics run counter to pessimistic pronouncements about an older woman's chances of success when it comes to pregnancy. That these often economically disadvantaged women, who had inadequate health care, and unfavorable circumstances, could have children[119] highlights not only a kind of tenacious quality about our biology, but specifically about our fertility at midlife as well.)

Contemporary women are mostly very different from their ancestors at age 35 and over and have great advantages when it comes to health risks in pregnancy.

More second and third babies are born to midlife women as a group, yet the rate of *first-time* mothers having babies in their mid-to late thirties and early forties has continued to increase.[120] The mothers in these age groups are among the most educated of all women, as well as being more affluent.[121] Their affluence and education bring them the advantage of good health care, including attention to exercise and diet, and high use of prenatal care.[122] And becoming a mother is a *choice;* they are highly motivated to take the best care possible during their pregnancies, as their babies are usually very much wanted.

RISK: THE COMMONSENSE APPROACH

All these differences make a midlife woman's pregnancy today very different from such pregnancy in the past, and make a healthy pregnancy the experience of most women at 35 and over. Yet despite these advantages, in our middle years our bodies are simply older. Even though pregnancy problems are much more the exception than the rule, having a baby when older carries more risk. I lay this statement at the door of common sense because conclusions vary enormously within the community of medical researchers (whose work in turn informs and influences how your doctor cares for you).

Pregnancy-induced hypertension and gestational or maternal diabetes (you'll find brief descriptions of these conditions in the earlier section, "The Preconception Physical Exam") are among the most often mentioned pregnancy problems for older women, both in medical literature and by physicians. Here is a current sample of the breadth of views about risks.

These two pregnancy complications have been found to be *significantly* associated with pregnancies over 35 in one study,[123] yet in another, midlife subjects were *not* found to be at higher risk for preeclampsia or gestational diabetes.[124] While it seems obvious that the possibility of developing problems in pregnancy are minimized by starting out healthy regardless of a woman's age, according to another source, during gestation, complications that are not necessarily evident beforehand are more likely to crop up for older women.[125] Which source should you believe? Should you feel reassured or worried?

Further, there is a gap in the statistical orientation of a medical study versus a "clinical" one—that is, having to do with the direct experience of a clinician, that person being your doctor—that easily lends itself to some confusion. For instance, the term *significant* describing the statistical findings in a study conveys a tone of authority and great probability. It's easy to translate a phrase such as "significant association" or "significant increase" into "So large a number of women in our study, all pregnant at midlife *like you*, developed diabetes and hypertension, it's a good bet that you will too."

It is important to know, however, that statistical findings say much more about the experience of a *group* than they do about what your experience is or will be as an *individual*. Thoughtful physicians view applying group statistics directly to an individual patient as inappropriate and invalid. (Unfortunately, this distinction gets blurred in some medical practices and of course in popular media sources such as newspaper stories and television news.)

Here is the commonsense approach: Diabetes and hypertension are among the top three (anemia is the third) medical problems that develop in pregnancy for *all* age groups.[126] As mentioned earlier, age and weight heighten your chances of developing these conditions. Many of us fit the bill on both counts, having already gained a little or a lot of weight as the years went by. Being older, we are more likely to have chronic conditions that we take into pregnancy and that sometimes create problems. So, although healthy midlife women shouldn't expect any complications, probably we *are* more at risk with pregnancy over 35, and probably a little more so after 40.

MORE RISK IS NOT HIGH RISK

More risk in pregnancy, however, is different from a "high-risk pregnancy," a term that has been synonymous with midlife pregnancy until recently. In fact, many of the studies that do find a greater rate of complications for older women also conclude that, nevertheless, a midlife woman can still expect that she and her baby will be just fine.[127]

Garden-variety pregnancy problems (such as the top three mentioned above), although potentially serious and especially so if left untreated, are generally monitored by your ob/gyn. A high-risk pregnancy is one where a condition is present that clearly increases the possibility of complications for either mother or baby.[128] For instance, carrying triplets or a history of premature deliveries would indeed justify the monitoring and care provided by a perinatologist.

Age alone does not make an older woman's pregnancy precarious. However, if your physician is very conservative, believing that any increase in risk at all is justification enough, or if your physician simply is not current on the subject, a healthy 35-plus woman with no worrisome symptoms whatsoever might find herself in high-risk care.

If this is so for you, you can either take comfort in the extra scrutiny of your progress, or, if it is either too invasive or actually makes you fearful about your pregnancy, you can get a referral to a care provider whose approach is more compatible with yours. And keep in mind, although problems during pregnancy may be more of a possibility for older women as a group, as with the issue of subfertile versus infertile, risk is relative too; *more* risk does not mean *high* risk.

CESAREAN DELIVERIES AT 35-PLUS

Age *is* indisputably linked, however, with an increase in cesarean deliveries. Studies report women over 35 to be *six times* as likely as younger women to have cesarean births.[129] The question is, are those additional c-sections performed out of medical necessity or do they have more to do with a "physician factor"?

A "physician factor" may come into play if the choice of an operative delivery is based not on any real danger to mother or baby associated with a vaginal birth, but instead is based on the mother's age as the sole or primary consideration. Such a doctor need not be ready to operate at the drop of a hat; rather, he or she may have doubts about the capacity of older women in general to labor successfully, despite the lack of evidence for this point of view.

In fact, several studies implicate physician bias and suggest that many midlife women may be having unnecessary cesareans.[130] (Only one of the many reports I used for my research on pregnancy risks for older women concluded otherwise.[131]) For some obstetricians, even a mild condition that arises in an older woman during her pregnancy, labor, or delivery might warrant a cesarean,[132] for others, a c-section is a foregone conclusion for any woman over 35.[133]

Some doctors place "premium baby" status on midlife babies, especially those of 40-plus women, where it is more likely to be an only or last baby because of the fertility and time issue. While a physician with this viewpoint may also be more inclined to recommend a c-section when it's not entirely necessary, many women appreciate the heightened concern about the safety of their baby during labor. They just want their baby to be safe, and trust the doctor's assessment about the wisdom of a surgical rather than vaginal delivery.

Is a midlife woman more likely to have complications that warrant a cesarean delivery? The answer appears to be inconclusive and conflicting. Your best course of action, regardless of study conclusions, is to have a straightforward talk with your doctor about how he or she approaches cesarean deliveries. You want to know what pregnancy and labor problems are indications for c-sections. You want to know if they are performed more often with midlife patients, and if so, why? Ask if your doctor has any concerns that you may be headed for a cesarean birth, and why, and how that problem will be monitored or treated throughout your pregnancy.

After you've gathered information, if you feel strongly about not having an operative delivery, tell your doctor that although your safety and your baby's safety are absolutely the primary concern, you are aware that especially for women over 35, every cesarean is not a necessary cesarean. Clearly express that you want great care taken in assessing for medical necessity if a c-section becomes a possibility. (Even in a health care setting where the doctor or midwife who delivers your baby is the one who happens to be on duty at that time, and not necessarily your own obstetrician, you can still have this discussion. Get a sense of the general policy toward cesareans that are guidelines for all hospital staff.) Your obstetrician should be receptive to this kind of talk, and if not, this may be a sign you're working with the wrong doctor.

The chances are overwhelming that your doctor's focus is your safety during pregnancy and labor as well as the successful delivery of a healthy baby. Yet because it does appear that midlife women are more likely to have unnecessary surgical deliveries, it can only help for you to be direct with your questions and clear about your wishes.

As a middle-years woman, you are bound to be more informed—and thus more-worried—than a blissfully naive 20-year-old. While it will be to your advantage to make regular prenatal care appointments to catch as soon as possible any problems that do develop, the best approach is to be informed and watchful, but *justifiably* confident.

What you want in your ob/gyn is a physician who is informed about pregnancy risks for older women, who was thorough at your preconception exam, and who is watchful for the earliest signs of problems at your prenatal visits—but who, given your continued good health, is confident in your body's capacity to carry a pregnancy and deliver a baby safely and well.

DOWN SYNDROME—THE POSITIVE REALITY

Popular opinion about the hazards of midlife pregnancy is a mixed bag. Many of us have mothers or grandmothers who had their babies at midlife, or have heard stories about it in conversations with friends or even with a friendly stranger. It doesn't seem so unusual then, and the risks hardly notable if any are mentioned at all. Many others, however, have lingering fears inspired mostly by the increase in chromosomal abnormalities at 35 years, such as Down syndrome.[134]

Pregnancy at midlife does not carry great extra health risks for your baby. In fact, outside of the increase in chromosomal abnormalities, a healthy 35-plus woman without pregnancy complications is as likely as a younger woman to have a baby without medical problems.[135] And even when it comes to chromosomal disorders, *your chances of conceiving a baby with Down syndrome are actually very low.*

This is so even though the increase in chromosomal disorders associated with age is the one unquestionable health risk to your baby, *and* despite the fact that the increases over the years are enormous. Your chances of having a Down's baby as a 27-year-old woman are 1 in 1,111; at 37 it rises to 1 in 227, and then increases even further, to 1 in 50, at age 43.[136]

It is a rare woman who is able to totally dismiss the chromosomal issue and completely quiet her feelings of apprehension about her baby's health. The increases in occurrence represent a loss of security and comfort that is more often a part of being pregnant younger, when the odds are so excellent for a chromosomally normal baby. Worrying about Down syndrome is the only difficult part about midife pregnancy for many older women.

Some women are certain they would not terminate a Down syndrome pregnancy. Nevertheless, knowing a Down's baby is on the way requires a relinquishment of dreams involving a normal child, a shift in expectations, and practical preparations they didn't plan on when they decided to have a baby. For those who would consider an abortion, the "Down's issue" can mean everything: the possibility of terminating their pregnancy, dealing with all of the emotional aftermath, starting over. This is a difficult experience for most women of any age. But at midlife, especially in the late thirties and particularly into the forties, it is compounded by an additional layer of concern about time limits on fertility.

However, let's take a step back from the visceral impact of these numbers. At age 43, 1 in 50, or 2 in 100 women will conceive a baby with Down's. *This means that even at 43, your chances of having a baby* without *Down syndrome are 98 out of 100, or 98 percent.* Who of us would not take a wanted risk that offers a 98 percent chance of success? Your chances for a chromosomally normal baby at 27 are excellent, yet at 43 they are still very good. We will revisit this point in the chapter ahead on prenatal testing, again placing it in the rational, commonsense, positive perspective it should be viewed in when it comes to being pregnant at midlife.

The chromosomal issue is part of the reality of having a baby at midlife. It is a part of being pregnant in our middle years that many of us grapple with, either before or after we have conceived. Once pregnant, some women think about it on a daily basis, others only once in a while or maybe even just once before settling the issue firmly and putting it to rest. However you feel, keep in mind that your chance of having a perfectly healthy baby at midlife is part of the reality too.

TWO

A Preconception Shortcut

The preconception plan discussed in Chapter One will help you make the best start you can into pregnancy. You have taken care of any health concerns prepregnancy, and are now alert to those pre-existing medical conditions (if any) that need to be monitored during your pregnancy. You've discontinued drinking alcoholic beverages and using prescribed medications that might cause birth defects, and you are making sure you're taking in all the important nutrients to help create the healthiest conditions possible for both yourself and the baby. You now know how to identify your most fertile days, you've had a fertility check, and any problems uncovered are being dealt with. All the basics have been covered. (Refer back to Chapter One for a fuller walk through preconception preparations.)

Some midlife women, however, feel more than a little anxious about being able to get pregnant. Even when everything looks fine—the signs of ovulation are obvious, their cycles are normal— because of their age, they wonder if their eggs are still good enough to make a baby.

If you feel this way, or if you have an overwhelming sense of readiness and longing or otherwise just want more information *up front* about your chances for conceiving, there is one additional step you can take in doing your prepregnancy groundwork; you can have your egg quality tested.

A simple addition to the basic fertility check, this approach involves borrowing two test measures usually reserved for infertility patients to make an assessment of your egg quality. Tested on the third day of your cycle via a simple blood test, these are measurements of the reproductive hormones, called *follicle stimulating hormone,* or *FSH,* and *Estradiol,* or *E2.*[1]

Each of these hormones plays an important role in the process of ovulation,[2] and the levels of FSH and E2 in your blood give your doctor valuable information about the quality of your eggs.[3] Egg quality is not the only factor involved, but is the most significant one in evaluating your fertility.[4]

Medically speaking, a couple isn't considered infertile until they've been unable to conceive a child after twelve months of regular, unprotected intercourse. This definition is actually more of a treatment directive than a certain statement about your fertility; you may indeed be fertile, but simply take longer than a year to conceive. Nevertheless, as most women do conceive within twelve months, the standard of care by and large is to consult with your physician if you are not pregnant after a year has passed.

For women 35-plus, *six months* without conceiving is the time limit to keep in mind.[5] While there is no standard guideline specific to age 40 and over, according to some physicians, a woman should consider taking action if she is not pregnant within *three months.*[6] Why should a healthy 40-year-old run to the doctor after three months when a typical, fertile midlife woman may take *longer* to conceive than a woman in her twenties? Because of our reproductive time limits.

Testing your FSH and E2 early on might save you three to six months of precious time, or can offer something else valuable when you're uneasy about the state of your fertility—the reassurance of knowing that yes, my eggs are in good shape and yes, my chances for getting pregnant are probably pretty good. This is the sort of information that goes a long way toward helping you be more relaxed while waiting to conceive.

However, if your FSH and E2 levels indicate your egg quality to be borderline, you may decide to move on to a reproductive specialist relatively quickly to make full use of your current degree of fertility. This is the biggest advantage to testing your FSH and your E2 levels.

This shortcut approach runs counter to the "until proven otherwise" standard practiced in fertility medicine, whereby a woman's fertility is assumed and a fertility problem is "proven" to exist only when pregnancy doesn't happen according to the guidelines above. Certainly, on the face of it, this rule of thumb is positive, wise, and sensible; why undergo any sort of testing for infertility before demonstrating any infertility?

First, we should shift the focus and think of these as *fertility* rather than *infertility* tests. Second, while the chances are good that most midlife women wanting babies can have them, the older you are, the more likely you are to become not *sub*fertile but *in*fertile. Thus, there is less time to work with any fertility problems toward a successful pregnancy. Although this is especially so for women in their late thirties and beyond, when the limits on fertility are in all probability drawing near, preconception fertility testing makes good sense for *any* highly motivated midlife woman.

The disadvantages of these tests, however, are not insignificant. Your ob/gyn may not be familiar with FSH or E2 testing, or he or she may not place the premium value upon these assessments that up-to-date infertility specialists do. Your doctor may not only be reluctant to order these tests, but may also be inexperienced at interpreting your results.

If you encounter such resistance, you can ask for a referral to a reputable specialist. If you are referred "in-house," for instance, if you get your medical care through a health maintenance organization where referral from one department to another is customary, the costs of these tests will probably be covered. If you are referred to a specialist outside your HMO, however, chances are you will have to pay out of pocket, and not only for these tests, but for any infertility treatment that may follow.

Health insurance benefits that do include coverage for infertility may follow the "until proven otherwise" guidelines. If so, this means you must try to conceive on your own for the period of time stipulated in your particular policy (typically ranging from six months to two years) before any infertility care will be paid for. This is a huge practical factor in choosing whether to have your FSH and E2 tested early on. If you wish to move aggressively, make some inquiries into the extent of the ob/gyn care and infertility treatment allowed by your health plan, and what period of time must elapse (if any, as many but not all have a time requirement) for you to receive coverage. Explore the extent of your financial commitment as it can be significant.

The second thing to consider before you take these tests is the emotional risk, and you've probably already guessed it. These tests can indicate that your chances of getting pregnant with your own eggs could be slim to none. It is a terrible feeling when failure is predicted before you even try. It is a loss in and of itself because the process of trying to realize a most-wanted dream holds a great deal of meaning.

Some women, even when highly motivated to have a baby, simply do not want to take these tests because they're not ready to make what could be a devastating discovery so soon. For them, it is more important to let nature take its course. They prefer to try conceiving with the assumption that they are fertile.

The other option with negative FSH/E2 results is to consult an infertility specialist about his or her recommendations for you to become a mother. Although not your first choice, reproductive technology offers other possibilities to women when the quality of their eggs makes natural conception a longshot. Here, too, there are significant costs to consider.

THREE

Prenatal Testing: Embracing Your Pregnancy, Finally

Prenatal testing to diagnose or screen for genetic birth defects is a standard feature of middle-years pregnancy. Even if only as an option to decline, it is part of the package of issues to consider that comes with being pregnant today as a midlife woman.

But remember that having a baby does not suddenly become intrinsically risky at age 35. Rather, offering genetic testing to women at this age became the standard of care because of the greater risk of having a child with a chromosomal disorder, *and* because of a procedure-related risk factor: At age 35 the risk of having a baby with a chromosomal abnormality is equivalent to the risk of a miscarriage from amniocentesis (the rate for each is about 1 in 200).[1] As both pose the same small but significant risks, the choice of whether to have amniocentesis is up to you.

It is also important to understand the parameters of prenatal diagnosis. Testing cannot detect most birth defects,[2] and no test is 100 percent flawless in picking up detectable problems. Nor can testing reliably indicate the severity of a condition discovered in utero. Further, while chromosomal disorders and neural tube defects are routinely tested for, clinicians only check for genetic disorders such as Tay-Sachs, sickle cell anemia, thalassemia, muscular dystrophy, and cystic fibrosis when there is a confirmed risk based on prior testing.[3] For most of us in our middle years, however, prenatal diagnosis is about detecting chromosomal abnormalities, and specifically whether the baby has Down syndrome. (Down syndrome accounts for about half the chromosomal disorders found in the pregnancies of women 35 and over.[4]) Test results for this condition are better than 99 percent accurate.[5]

Most of us invest a lot of emotion in a wanted pregnancy. Even just conceiving can unleash a whole array of intense feelings and fantasies. As time goes by, the sense of being a pregnant woman grows. You identify yourself as a mother-to-be; a connection that began with the simple awareness that a tiny fetus now exists in your belly deepens into a relationship with "the baby" long before it is born. No wonder, then, that many women approach prenatal diagnosis with a blend of fear and anticipation.

A woman having a second trimester prenatal diagnosis procedure has had weeks and months for her emotions to build. The day of the test may loom large, like a giant question mark hanging over the course of her pregnancy. Testing is a definite crossroads for a woman certain she'd terminate a Down syndrome pregnancy. Up until now, there has probably been some degree of *splitting* in how she felt about having a baby. She may have held back some of the joy, deflected away some of her fantasies of what this child might be like, hidden a part of her heart away in case she might have to decide to let go.

At the same time, she has done all she can to protect and care for her baby in utero, eaten as well as possible, taken prenatal vitamins, avoided exposure to anything that has even a remote possibility of being toxic, thought *soft* over *cute* when doing some early browsing for baby clothes.

For a woman positive she would not have an abortion, the prenatal diagnosis is still a landmark, providing information that gives her a chance to make special preparations in advance, if need be. And for a woman less sure about having an abortion, and uncertain of her feelings about raising a child with a disability, this point can be something of a crucible, forcing her to make a difficult decision. Whichever point of view is yours, if you choose to have prenatal diagnosis testing means that the question, "Does my baby have Down syndrome?" will be answered.

Those who decide to continue with their pregnancies are now freed of uncertainty. They can stop splitting their feelings; they can fully glory in being pregnant women, they can totally thrill in feeling the baby kick or hiccup, imagine holding their son or daughter for the first time. In other words, these women can finally and fully embrace their pregnancy.

The next section takes a look at the five most widely used prenatal tests to diagnose and screen for genetic abnormalities; amniocentesis, chorionic villus sampling, alpha fetoprotein screening, multiple marker screening, and ultrasound. Most of these are routinely offered to midlife women as part of their prenatal care. Finding out whether your developing baby has particular birth defects relatively early in pregnancy is on the whole a real advantage. However, all these tests offer a mixture of benefits, risks, and drawbacks.

An ideal prenatal test would be an early, noninvasive, accurate procedure, with results that are ready quickly. Unfortunately, the "perfect" test is not yet available. Chorionic villus sampling (CVS), although not recommended before your tenth week, can be performed relatively early in pregnancy. Yet test results take up to three weeks. In the best circumstances, a woman gets her results in barely enough time to make a first trimester abortion possible. Both CVS and amniocentesis offer accurate results but are invasive procedures. Multiple marker screening (MMS), while requiring only a blood sample, does not offer the accuracy of CVS and amniocentesis.

I'll describe the pros and cons of each of the five tests in more detail below. Understanding the advantages and disadvantages involved in having a test is especially important when it comes to making a decision about amniocentesis and CVS, the two diagnostic procedures that carry small but known risks to the fetus.

But first, a thought to carry with you while reading about these tests. Although most pregnant women of *any* age worry about their baby's health, considering prenatal diagnosis or screening magnifies these worries tenfold. You can be plagued by the thought that a birth defect is out there with your baby's name on it, and even come to feel that having a normal, perfect child is a rarity.

This feeling is the natural outgrowth of being informed and educated about the risks. Rather than putting a lot of energy into repressing it, you may be more comfortable acknowledging your fears, and at the same time acknowledging that the odds of having a normal baby are still very, very much in your favor at midlife. Even at 45, your chance of not having a baby with Down syndrome is better than 96 percent.[6]

Amniocentesis

Mid-trimester amniocentesis is the gold standard of prenatal diagnosis. It provides the most information, most accurately, with the least risk to you or your baby. It detects better than 99 percent of chromosomal disorders and over 90 percent of neural tube defects (NTDs).[7] (Remember that the incidence of NTDs is *not* age-related. You are no more likely to have a baby with this type of birth defect at midlife than you were as a woman of 18 or 20.) The risks of a test-related miscarriage, a primary concern with any invasive procedure for prenatal diagnosis, is low. For mid-trimester (also called "standard") amniocentesis, it is about 1 in 200. Some believe it may be as low as 1 in 400,[8] because of the years of experience many physicians have accumulated in performing this test, as well as the now-common practice of using ultrasound guidance throughout the entire procedure.

Amniocentesis is performed as you lie on an examining table. Before the actual procedure, an ultrasound exam will confirm the age of the fetus, the location of both the fetus and the placenta, and whether there is sufficient quantity of amniotic fluid for the sample needed to conduct the lab tests that will follow.

The physician uses the ultrasound image as a guide to safely avoid the fetus and placenta. After cleaning the area with an antiseptic solution, the physician inserts a slender needle through your abdominal wall and the uterus into the amniotic sac, drawing a small amount of amniotic fluid. Analysis of the amniotic fluid will answer a number of questions about your baby.

Within one day after conception, the embryo divides into two cells, and by four days, it multiplies to become sixteen tiny cells all together in a cluster. At five or six days a major development takes place when the cells of the embryo rearrange to form an inner and an outer layer. The outer layer of cells will implant in the uterine wall, becoming part of the placenta; those on the inside will become a baby. Both the baby and the placenta (in part) develop from egg and sperm.[9]

The baby growing inside the amniotic sac is cushioned and supported by the fluid that fills it. (Early in pregnancy the mother's fluid is the main source for amniotic fluid, and after about twenty weeks, it comes mostly from the urine put out by the fetus.[10]) The developing baby makes a substance called *alpha-fetoprotein*, or *AFP*, that is found in the amniotic fluid. The level of AFP can be tested to detect neural tube disorders.

Spina bifida, where the spinal cord is exposed,[11] and *anencephaly*, involving abnormal development in both the brain and head, are the two most common NTDs.[12] These defects are thought to result from a combination of genetic and environmental causes. One to two babies per 1,000 in North America are born with spina bifida.[13] AFP is present in fetal blood as well as in the mother's blood, where the amount can also be checked with a separate test called *alpha fetoprotein screening*, or a test known as *multiple marker screening*.[14] Both of these tests will be discussed later in this chapter.

Amniotic fluid also contains cells the developing baby has shed and therefore can reveal the baby's genetic makeup. The cells will be analyzed for chromosomal abnormalities. The baby's sex can be determined by studying the chromosomes as well. Lab results can take up to three weeks.[15]

Amniocentesis is usually done during the first month of the second trimester, at fifteen to eighteen weeks.[16] (Pregnancy is dated from the first day of your last menstrual period, or LMP, even when you are absolutely certain of the day you conceived!) After fifteen weeks, the chances are good that there will be sufficient amniotic fluid and enough fetal cells present to successfully run the necessary lab tests.

This procedure can be done earlier than fifteen weeks as well as later than eighteen weeks. However, at eighteen-*plus* weeks, if a problem is detected and a woman wants the option of terminating her pregnancy, timing becomes an issue. Typically, twenty-one weeks is the limit to have an abortion in a clinic setting rather than in a hospital, and twenty-four weeks is the latest point abortions may be performed in many medical facilities.[17] Since lab results take up to three weeks, and occasionally a test must be repeated if the first attempt doesn't work (because of glitches in the lab testing process, for instance), having an amniocentesis beyond eighteen weeks may run you beyond those time restrictions.

⅖ Early Amniocentesis

Amniocentesis performed earlier than fifteen weeks is called *early amniocentesis.* The procedure is the same as for standard amniocentesis, but simply takes place before the fifteenth week of pregnancy. A few have been done at ten to eleven weeks, more and more are being performed at twelve to thirteen weeks, but most often early amniocentesis is done during a woman's fourteenth week.[18]

Early amniocentesis offers the possibility of learning if the fetus has a chromosomal abnormality before the first fetal movements are felt, which usually occurs between sixteen and twenty weeks.[19] This is an important factor in choosing a prenatal test for women who would consider an abortion, depending on their test results. For many, feeling movement generates the first real sense that something alive is within their body; along with this comes a deepening connection to the developing baby. The process of considering an abortion if the fetus is found to have a major birth defect is less wrenching before this much development has taken place.

Feelings about early amniocentesis are mixed in the medical community. For starters, the rate of miscarriage may be as high as 2.5 times that of the standard test.[20] This procedure is performed relatively rarely, and therefore medical professionals have less information about this test than either standard amniocentesis or chorionic villus sampling.[21] For instance, while a woman's body produces enough amniotic fluid to draw from and there are adequate fetal cells at this point to productively study and analyze in the lab—early amino is now believed to be as accurate as standard amnio[22]—there is some uncertainty as to the wisdom of puncturing the amnion—the membrane covering the inside of the amniotic sac—so soon.[23] You may want to talk about these concerns with your doctor in deciding whether to have early amniocentesis.

Physician experience is *most* important when it comes to a safe, successful amniocentesis, either standard or early. You will want to make some inquiries about your clinician's level of experience as well as his or her reputation. The experience should be a matter of record openly discussed with you when you ask.

Speak directly with the physician, the nurse, or genetics personnel involved in patient care and ask:

1. How many years have/has you/the doctor been doing amnios?

2. How many do you/they perform annually? Monthly? (Your best bet is a clinician who stays practiced on a consistent basis throughout the year.)

3. Have any of your patients lost pregnancies following an amnio you performed? How many? (Their procedure-related loss rate should be *no higher* than the average of one miscarriage per 200 amnios.)

The State of California Department of Health Services has now established standards for state-approved prenatal diagnosis centers.[24] Among many requirements for both the centers and their physicians, each practitioner must have completed 100 supervised, ultrasound-guided standard amnios, and thereafter must perform 50 or more per year.

A too-high *adverse outcome rate* for an individual physician practicing in a state-approved prenatal diagnosis center, that is when there are more procedure-related miscarriages than is usually associated with amniocentesis, must be reported to the department's Genetic Disease Branch by either the physician or the facility at which he or she performs the procedure.[25] Additionally, each physician is monitored about once every five years for the overall outcome of the procedures performed.[26] All this information on both performance and results must be relayed to the state in order to maintain state approval. The outcome for *all* early amnios must also be submitted.

To be approved for early amniocentesis, 10 of the initial 100 supervised amnios may actually be early instead of standard amnios; that is, done prior to fifteen weeks rather than at fifteen weeks or later. Performing an *additional* ten procedures within the twelve- to fifteen-week time frame for early amniocentesis is an option for approval. Also, clinicians approved for standard amniocentesis whose experience with the early procedure predates January 1, 1996, are grandfathered in. This date marks the point when the standards for physicians performing early amniocentesis in approved prenatal diagnosis centers were set.

Check in your state for any physician standards regarding am-

niocentesis (and chorionic villus sampling). Your state's health services department is a good starting point. If not, California's
standards can at least offer some guidelines. The Genetic Disease
Branch of the Department of Health Services in California can be
contacted at (510) 540–2534 for information about the requirements
for centers. California residents can also get locations of approved
centers and the names of approved physicians.

Whether or not you are having your amniocentesis in a medical
clinic or institution that is certified as described above, you will still
want to do some checking on your own to find the physician on staff
with the best reputation for performing this procedure. Even among
a group of qualified practitioners, one or more are likely to be *quietly*
known for their technical skill. (It's unlikely that any medical professional you speak with will *openly* rate colleagues.)

Although reputations most certainly can be built without any
worthy foundation, often enough you can gather some useful information despite the subjectivity involved. If you receive your
medical care in a setting where more than one doctor does the
amnios, you may want to speak privately with various medical
staff. Ask a favorite nurse: Who is the best at amniocentesis? Who
would you want if you needed one? Who would you want your
daughter to have do hers?

If your choice is limited to one physician, you might ask:
Would Dr. X be your first choice to do an amnio on you, or is
there another physician you'd ask first? Would Dr. X be your first
choice to do your daughter's, or is there another physician you'd
go to first? If you are not totally reassured by the response you
get, make inquiries about other places you could go in your city.

HAVING AN AMNIOCENTESIS

The overall physical process of having an amniocentesis has
two prominent features: the needle insertion itself, and the sensation of an (overly!) full bladder. Although it's not always required,[27] some physicians direct their patients to drink as much as

four cups of water just prior to their appointment time in preparation for the pre-amnio ultrasound. Many women actually find this to be the more difficult experience of the two!

The experience of having a needle inserted through your abdomen and into the uterus is different for everyone. Your doctor can numb the area with an injection beforehand, but some women find this even more uncomfortable than the procedure itself. In fact, although it is painful for some women, most are surprised at how little if any discomfort they felt.[28] Imagining the worst, plus the long buildup to the day of the test, maybe seeing the needle beforehand, can all add to any discomfort you may feel.

To help you handle the perfectly natural and common fears and anxiety you may experience, here are some thoughts:

- Know that you *can* do this. Other women have done it before you; you *too* have the capacity to see this procedure through.

- Remind yourself that you very much want a child, and that this is part of the process you feel you need to go through to have that baby.

- Remember that you have minimized the risks that come with amniocentesis by finding the best physician you could to perform yours.

- Tell yourself that you'd rather go through this process, however formidable, than be surprised by the birth of a child with a severe abnormality.

- If you miscarried a previous pregnancy before your amnio was scheduled, celebrate the fact that you are now far enough along to be having this procedure.

WAITING

If I could design the ideal test for prenatal diagnosis, the waiting period for receiving the results would be somewhere between an hour and a day. On one hand, even though the chance there is a problem is a small one, the possibility of learning on the spot that my baby had a major birth defect might be a bit much to psychologically prepare for on top of gearing up for the procedure itself. I wonder if most of us wouldn't need at least a little time for the test to first be over before we go on to the next step of getting ourselves ready to receive the results. On the other hand, spending many days or a period of weeks wondering and worrying is, to say the least, uncomfortable.

When you have an amniocentesis, although it is not uncommon to get test results in ten to twelve days, many patients can expect to wait two to three weeks.[29] The time it takes depends for the most part on how quickly the fetal cells from the amniotic fluid sample taken during your amniocentesis are growing. The waiting can be difficult to endure precisely because the test outcome matters so much.

This is a good time to take it easy, emotionally. Be gentle with yourself, and nurture yourself in whatever ways work best for you. Your goal is simply to make it through these next few days or weeks as comfortably as you can.

Read books that take your thoughts away from your own concerns, or let yourself be distracted from them by becoming immersed in a project. Take unhurried walks. Sit in a garden or go to the beach and watch the waves. Watch your favorite movies. Get a massage or a facial. Take a day trip with your husband. Speak with good friends about what you are feeling and your worries about the test—or not. Either way, bask in the support of those friendships. If intense anxiety grips you, purposefully slow your breath, shifting your attention to the rhythm of your breathing until you feel more relaxed, even if only for a few moments.

One of my midlife clients spent an hour or so at the beach near her home every day while she was waiting for the results of her amniocentesis. Said Debra, "My best friend's brother had Down syndrome. His problems were severe, and while I admired how well they did as a family, I knew I would not choose to start out as a mother with a severely disabled child.

"I was definitely on edge about my test results. Every time I'd think about it—several times per day—I'd feel very anxious. My daily walks really helped. The movement of the water was soothing, the warmth of the sun and smells from the ocean were pleasant—it all seemed to make that time pass more easily. I still find that the beach soothes me, but of course the pleasure is many times greater now when I walk there with my healthy young daughter."

For Marian, remaining busy and involved with work was helpful. She even planned her amniocentesis for the week before an out-of-state conference she and her husband would be attending together. Marian explains, "If I was home, I would be unable to keep myself from literally waiting by the phone every day until I heard the results of my test. I knew that getting out of town, negotiating around an unfamiliar city, participating in meetings and events would serve as a distraction from my thoughts. I was also happy that I would be doing all that with my husband. I believe bearing the uncertainty of not knowing what the results would be while we were together in this way made it easier for both of us.

"It turned out to be the best conference either of us ever went to. Partway through it, I received a message that my doctor needed to speak with me. Since it was now only ten days after I'd had the procedure, we hadn't really expected the test results to come back so quickly. We imagined there might be some terrible news waiting for us that our doctor felt we should know as soon as possible. But when we immediately called back, the news was good! No Down syndrome, no spina bifida—everything looked great! We were relieved and just ecstatic."

For some women, the combination of distraction and nurturance fits their lives best. Janet worked full-time, but let her household task schedule slip while she was waiting. Instead, she made sure she had ninety minutes of free time each evening. "I'd read books or watch

TV or speak on the phone with close friends. I felt lucky that two of them had gone through prenatal testing when they were pregnant, one at 37 and the other at 40. Their understanding of just what it was like to wait to find out if the baby was normal or not was incredibly supportive. Other times I'd just sit quietly with a cup of tea; I'd do whatever felt good to me that night.

"While I was too busy at work to dwell for long on my fears about the test results, the ever-present underlying worry was emotionally wearing. Taking it extra easy every night helped me replenish myself in preparation for the next day of work, and waiting. The days seemed to drag by, but once the genetic counselor called eighteen days later, upon hearing that the tests showed my baby boy was chromosomally normal, even the memory of the angst I'd carried around for nearly three weeks simply vanished."

There is no way to avoid going through this waiting period unless you choose not to have amniocentesis, or CVS. Though the vast, vast majority of test results are good, no one should expect you to pass through this time without being anxious. It's okay to feel anxious. The best course is to take good care of yourself and let those who love you know how they can help.

Amniocentesis is still not quite an ideal pregnancy test on another count. Both the early and standard procedures take place within the second trimester, meaning that if need be, a second trimester abortion would be necessary to terminate the pregnancy.

A pregnancy terminated in your first trimester between six and thirteen weeks, with either an *aspiration* abortion or by *dilation and curettage*, or *D&C*, involves a much safer and simpler procedure than the one performed between thirteen and twenty-four weeks. In your second trimester, a *dilation and evacuation*, or *D&E*, typically involves a two-day procedure. Further, most doctors recommend a hospital rather than a clinic setting for a D&E done after twenty-one weeks.[30]

The uterus is softer and there is more fetal tissue in your second trimester than there is in your first. Thus, this is a procedure that requires more skill to safeguard against complications, such as perforating the uterus or overlooking fetal tissue in the evacuation process. If you need to have a D&E, by sure to inquire about the experience level and reputation of the clinician performing the procedure.

MAKING A DECISION ABOUT AMNIOCENTESIS

The decision to have amniocentesis rests with you. A midlife woman concerned about having a baby with a chromosomal disorder must weigh the benefit of knowing for sure against the risk of miscarriage. When it comes to making a decision about prenatal testing, the essential question is this: What is the risk worth to me? Is the small but documented possibility of a miscarriage worth knowing if the baby has Down syndrome? Some of my clients put it to themselves this way: Is it more important to me to continue this pregnancy and be a mother to this baby no matter what? Or would I rather know about chromosomal or other problems now, even if it means risking a miscarriage of a healthy baby?

Some pregnant midlife women believe that their current pregnancy is their last chance for a baby, and for some that may be true. For those unwilling, or very reluctant, to risk a miscarriage, or those who are simply turned off by the whole idea of amniocentesis for other reasons, but would still like some information about the health of the developing baby, there are options. These noninvasive screening tests do not offer the accuracy of amniocentesis, but may appeal to a woman with this point of view. Before we go into more detail about them, and how they might be useful to midlife women, let's look first at chorionic villus sampling.

Chorionic Villus Sampling

Chorionic villus sampling can be done either *transabdominally,* as with amniocentesis, or *transcervically.* The transcervical (TC-CVS) route involves carefully guiding a catheter through the vagina and cervix to the area where the placenta is developing between the inner wall of the uterus and the chorion (the outer membrance of the amniotic sac). The placenta begins as microscopic projections of tissue that extend from the surface of the chorion, connect with the uterine wall, and become established in the mother's blood supply.[31] Called *chorionic villi*, this tissue develops from the fertilized egg and thus shares the baby's genetic makeup.[32] Analyzing the sample of chorionic villi taken through CVS will reveal chromosomal abnormalities, as well as the sex of the baby. Neural tube defects cannot be detected with CVS. (You can have your alpha fetoprotein screened for NTDs separately.)

Transabdominal CVS (TA-CVS) differs only in that a needle is inserted through your abdomen to reach the chorionic villi. (This part is similar to amniocentesis, but then villi rather than amniotic fluid is withdrawn for testing.) Both the transabdominal and transcervical techniques take place (or should!) with ultrasound guidance.

The waiting period for CVS test results are the same as for amniocentesis, up to three weeks.[33] For thoughts about waiting out those days, see the earlier section on waiting for the results of your amnio.

CVS offers a woman wanting prenatal diagnosis a mixed bag of some real advantages along with risks she should look at carefully. The early timing of the test in the first trimester, and the possibility of avoiding a needle inserted through your abdomen if a transcervical CVS is preformed, are pluses. However, the slightly higher rate of procedure-related miscarriage, along with the possibility of causing limb abnormalities in the developing baby, make the decision to have CVS rather than amniocentesis a complex one for many women.

MISCARRIAGE AND CVS

The rate of miscarriage caused by CVS ranges from 1 in 200, up to 2 in 100, slightly higher than the 1 in 400 to 1 in 200 range for standard, mid-trimester amniocentesis.[34] Physician experience is thought to be an important factor in CVS-related miscarriage, as is experience in *both* the transcervical and transabdominal techniques.[35] There are those who believe that when your clinician is experienced at both types of CVS procedures, the increase in risk over standard amniocentesis ranges from none to small enough to be considered statistically insignificant.[36] Under certain conditions transabdominal CVS is considered less likely to cause a miscarriage than transcervical CVS. TA-CVS, however, is also associated with a higher percentage of limb abnormalities (more to follow on this). Obviously, the decisions you'll have to make with regard to this test aren't easy ones.

Most pregnancy losses happen within the first twelve weeks, although the majority are by the tenth week of gestation, the earliest point CVS is usually done. Hence, it is difficult to be certain that a woman who loses her pregnancy after CVS would not have miscarried even without the procedure. Nevertheless, for some women the timeliness CVS offers over standard amniocentesis is weighed against the fact that a precious pregnancy ends more often via this procedure.

For other women, however, reports about birth defects that may be caused by CVS cause even greater concern.

BIRTH DEFECTS AND CVS

Birth defects linked to CVS first became news in the early 1990s.[37] Reports about the effects of this procedure from two small samples of patients included severe limb deficiencies, such as missing or underdeveloped fingers and toes, in otherwise normal babies. Although there were other procedure-related birth defects, such as abnormal jaws and tongues,[38] the medical community has focused more attention and concern on the incidence of these limb reduction defects.

Several larger subsequent studies have also found that CVS does place a baby at higher risk for damage to tiny developing limbs; a small increase—about three more babies per 10,000 above the number that occur in the general population—was found over-all in a multicenter review of more than 39,000 women who had CVS.[39] (Some of the health care centers that contributed their statistics to this report had much higher rates than others.) However, another review, this one of 138,000 procedures, did not find the incidence of these limb reduction deficiencies (LRDs) to be greater than the rate in the non-CVS exposed general population.[40]

Reports such as this one have bolstered the confidence of physicians, genetic counselors, and others who support the use of CVS as a routine first trimester procedure for prenatal diagnosis. Their confidence is effectively passed on to their patients. Many pregnant women have chosen CVS, convinced that their babies are in little danger from the test and that any risk that does exist is a small one.[41] (Around 200,000 procedures were documented worldwide between 1983 and 1995.[42])

In fact, although not a consensus point of view, some physicians have arrived at the conclusion that CVS is safe under *certain conditions*: when CVS is done after your tenth week of pregnancy, and when a clinician experienced with the procedure performs the test. In other words, the *timing* of the test—considered the most critical factor—current theories suggest that prior to ten weeks fetal limb development is disrupted by CVS—along with *clinician experience* (as with procedure-caused miscarriage), may be crucial in minimizing the possibility of test-related birth defects.[43]

Yet the certainty of some CVS supporters[44] represents only one point in the range of opinions and beliefs about the test's potential for causing birth defects.[45] The fact that small increases have been found in procedures done by apparently experienced clinicians, and even when done at the ten-week mark,[46] creates an understandable sense of unease.

With so much at stake, sorting through the ambiguity engendered by these contrasting conclusions can be one of the more challenging tasks of midlife pregnancy. With more women than ever having children after 35, it's of greater concern than ever before.

Certainly for a woman leaning toward CVS, the scale of the

positive outcome studies can be a big help in providing the substantive evidence she needs to decide that CVS is a medically responsible choice.

ON THE FENCE ABOUT CVS

For those women who are less certain CVS is the right choice for them, however, the contrast in reports can complicate their decision about which (if any) prenatal test to have. For some women there is another problem: As yet there is no clear and consistent *explanation* for either set of reports about the links between CVS and limb abnormalities.

If you are on the fence about CVS, the following section may be useful to you, as it looks at some facts about this procedure in more detail. However, if you are already certain that CVS would be your choice for prenatal diagnosis, you may find this rather step-by-step approach redundant. If so, skip ahead to read about alpha fetoprotein screening.

Here is a quick walk through two possible explanations considered in recent studies conducted on procedure-related birth defects. Again, one has to do with the experience level of the physician, and the other with the timing of the test.

Some believe that physician experience is extremely important in regard to CVS-related birth defects,[47] while others question how crucial it is.[48] (This is in contrast to the issue of procedure-related miscarriage where there is more of a consensus that experience does count.)

A related issue is the question of whether transcervical CVS is safer than transabdominal CVS, or vice versa. Some physicians believe TA-CVS is associated with a higher rate of limb defects.[49] Although the numbers are low, 2.2 affected babies out of 10,000 TC-CVS procedures were found in one study, but nearly 6 in 10,000 of those tested with TA-CVS, about two and a half times as many.[50]

Transabdominal CVS is easier to learn than the transcervical method, and has some procedural similarities to amniocentesis. However, it does require greater technical skill than amniocentesis (a test more doctors are practiced at); there is the possibility that TA-CVS procedures are being performed by inexperienced doctors mistakenly confident because of their proficiency with amniocentesis.[51] The result could be more TA-CVS exposed babies with birth defects.

Gestational age, or the week of pregnancy the test is performed, is the factor linked to limb abnormalities most consistently. While unfortunately this link does not explain every case—for instance, one of the original alarming reports included birth defects associated with CVS done just *before* as well as *into* the *eleventh* week of pregnancy[52]—it seems to be a reasonable one. The recommendation that CVS be done no earlier than ten weeks appears to substantially reduce the possibility of procedure-related LRDs.[53]

Despite the ambiguity of the study findings, it also seems reasonable to believe that experience does indeed matter. In fact, not surprisingly, having your CVS done by an experienced clinician is one of the two most frequent recommendations made in reports on the risks of CVS.[54] (The other, of course, is that the test should be timed no earlier than the tenth week of pregnancy dated from the first day of your last menstrual period.)

What makes an experienced clinician when it comes to CVS? Although 100 per year has been suggested as the minimum for a practitioner to maintain procedural skills[55], the standards for physicians practicing in a state-approved prenatal diagnosis center (in California) require fewer (in part due to the concern that enough clinicians be available to do CVS).

To meet these standards, a physician who performs transcervical CVS must have completed a minimum of thirty procedures. At least five of those must be on women who plan on continuing their pregnancies regardless of the test results, where followup is possible. These five must be supervised by an ob/gyn experienced in TC-CVS. Practitioners who do transabdominal CVS must have performed no fewer than twenty-five procedures. Again at least five must be on women who plan to continue their pregnancies no matter what their test outcome might be, and must be supervised by an ob/gyn experienced in TA-CVS.[56]

To *retain* their approved status, these physicians must perform only a total of twenty-five of either the TA or TC procedures,[57] all on women who plan to give birth.[58] (This revision to California's guidelines was made in 1997.) The drop in numbers needed is due to the fact that a limited number of women want CVS and thus there are a limited number of ob/gyns who perform thirty transcervical or twenty-five transabdominal CVS procedures per year.[59] That fewer are then required is not ideal. However, these physicians must continue to participate in the monitoring and reporting process that goes along with practicing in a state-approved center.

MAKING A DECISION ABOUT CVS

The phrase "patient responsibility" takes on a new dimension in the decision to choose CVS. Unfortunately, consensus about the relationship between CVS and limb abnormalities may be years away.

Without a consensus in the medical community to rely on, deciding if the advantages of CVS outweigh the drawbacks falls heavily on your shoulders, much more so than is usual in making a weighty medical decision. Thus, an understanding of the benefits and risks involved is essential, as is sorting through them to clarify your priorities. A purposeful decision will leave you feeling most comfortable with whatever choice you make.

The following will help you consider your own feelings about the pros and cons. First is a summary of the most important points about CVS in comparison to amniocentesis. Second is a series of questions.

As you read through them, notice which ones evoke immediate answers. Although your answers may certainly change as you have a chance to thoroughly mull over the options or to simply go with what you feel, your initial uncensored responses may provide you with surprising self-knowledge about what matters most to you when it comes to prenatal diagnosis.

Summary: CVS versus Amniocentesis

MAJOR ADVANTAGES

1. *Timeliness.* CVS is a first trimester procedure, usually done at ten to twelve weeks[60] and therefore:

Before you feel fetal movement.

Before you've developed a deeper, months-long connection with the developing baby.

Before your pregnancy is showing.

If you decide to have an abortion based on abnormal test results, CVS allows for the possibility of terminating a pregnancy with a D&C rather than with a more difficult second trimester procedure. You can have CVS at ten weeks, leaving sufficient time for test results to come back (up to three weeks) and still make the cutoff point for a D&C (thirteen weeks). Check on the time limit in your area.

Even if you know you wouldn't terminate your pregnancy, CVS would allow you a little more time to adjust, gather information, and make the preparations involved in caring for a child with a disability or terminal illness. You would have more time to make any psychological preparations you may need for handling the baby's condition when your pregnancy becomes public.

2. *Comfort.* Transabdominal CVS is not painful for most women, but like amniocentesis, may be uncomfortable. Some women experience transcervical CVS as hardly more uncomfortable than a Pap smear, yet for others it can be quite painful.[61] Nevertheless, the idea of having a needle inserted through your belly is simply objectionable to some women, and they view TC-CVS as a more desirable alternative.

MAJOR DISADVANTAGES

1. *Higher rate of miscarriage* than with standard amniocentesis. Loss rates in comparison to early amnio range from slightly less to slightly more.[62]

2.   *Unexplained reports and conflicting study results* about an association between CVS and limb reduction defects.

3.   *Neural tube defects cannot be detected* with CVS. They require a blood test screening AFP levels between fifteen and twenty weeks.[63]

4.   *Sufficient time* must remain following a positive pregnancy test. For instance, cervical cultures are usually required beforehand, as certain infections could be harmful if introduced into the uterus via the TC-CVS procedure.[64] Time must be allowed for the cultures to grow and be analyzed.

5.   *Availability*. Fewer physicians are trained to perform chorionic villus sampling,[65] thus not all medical facilities offer it, especially those outside metropolitan areas.

QUESTIONS

1.   What is my *level of comfort* with the possibility of a procedure-related miscarriage? The questions below will help you clarify your answer:

- Is *any* risk a reasonable trade-off for the information this test will provide me?

- Is a *small* risk worth taking for this information?

- Am I comfortable with the degree of risk after I've learned all I can about my practitioner's track record and found it to be excellent? (As with amniocentesis, you should ask the number of pregnancy losses and the number of babies born with limb defects above the norm subsequent to their procedures. Ask how many years the physician has been doing both TG *and* CVS, TA-CVS the number performed annually, and roughly the number done per month.)

2.   What is my *level of comfort* with the possibility of limb defects caused by CVS?

- Is *any* risk at all a reasonable trade-off for the advantages CVS offers over amniocentesis?

- Is a *small* risk worth the possibility of a lifelong birth defect?

- Am I comfortable with the risk after I've learned all I can about my practitioner's track record and found it to be excellent?

3.   Do I want *any* decision-making about prenatal diagnosis to be part of my pregnancy?

- Am I comfortable with the possibility of raising a child with a disability, be it minor or major?

- Am I comfortable with the possibility of having a child with a terminal disorder?

- Is minimizing my attachment, or temporarily withholding my connection to my developing baby a loss I'm unwilling to take? Put another way, am I unwilling to do anything less than to totally and immediately embrace my pregnancy?

Halfway through these questions, you may have realized that you knew whether or not you will have CVS, or perhaps this list has served to confirm a decision already made beforehand. But if neither is the case for you—and being undecided is a perfectly reasonable place to be when it comes to something as important as prenatal diagnosis—your best course is to take as much time as your gestational age and prenatal diagnosis procedure timetable will allow you in making up your mind about CVS.

It is not necessarily easy to sort through the advantages and disadvantages of a medical procedure, especially one that remains controversial within the medical community. You may want to speak with a knowledgeable, experienced genetics counselor for help in weighing your individual risk of having a baby with Down syndrome against the risks and benefits of CVS, or either standard or early amniocentesis.

The questions above about weighing risk have to do with a generic age factor, the fact that the risk of chromosomal abnormalities becomes not high, but higher for *all* midlife women. However, *individual* circumstances can very much increase the possibility of conceiving, for instance, a baby with an inherited genetic disorder. When both the mother and father are carriers of the gene causing Tay-Sachs disease or sickle cell anemia, the chances are 25 percent that their child will have that disease, or 50 percent that their child will be a carrier.[66] In such cases weighing the added risk of having an affected child against the benefits would be an important additional consideration. Again, consulting with a genetics counselor can be very helpful when you are weighing several factors that could cause birth defects against the potential hazards involved in prenatal diagnosis testing.

Last, give your indecision words—talk about it with your husband and with trusted friends. Or, if it suits you better, mull over your thoughts without putting them into spoken words. Even if you are highly ambivalent about CVS at this point, you *will* come to a decision you are comfortable with, and make the choice that is the right one for you.

Let's take a look now at alpha fetoprotein screening, multiple marker screening, and ultrasound. These prenatal tests can help you individualize your risk of carrying a baby with chromosomal disorders such as Down syndrome, and certain other birth defects.

Alpha Fetoprotein Screening

Alpha fetoprotein is a substance found in a pregnant woman's blood and in the amniotic fluid. Women who have had CVS can take a blood test for AFP screening, as there is none in the tissue sample taken during that procedure. Women who have decided against amniocentesis, or women for whom prenatal diagnosis is not part of their routine prenatal care, as is the case most often for women younger than 35, will probably also be offered this blood test.

AFP screening is different from a diagnostic test that determines the actual presence of a birth defect. As a screening test, it gives an estimate of the level of risk for certain disorders.

This blood test is reliable only between fifteen and twenty weeks, with sixteen to seventeen weeks being the best time.[67] Targeting these weeks provides for a pregnancy mistakenly dated later than it really is, and allows a woman the choice of terminating her pregnancy if testing indicates a chromosomal problem. (Many facilities do not perform abortions beyond twenty-four weeks. Check the limit in your area.) This test primarily screens for neural tube disorders, but can also detect abdominal wall defects and some Down syndrome pregnancies (see below).

A higher than normal amount of AFP, called a *positive high*, may be a sign of a problem with the fetus, such as a neural tube defect. Less than normal, or a *positive low*, may be a sign of Down syndrome. Results are usually ready within two weeks.[68]

There is, unfortunately, a significant false negative rate, where test results are normal when in fact there is a birth defect. Only about 20 percent of Down syndrome pregnancies will be found through alpha fetoprotein screening, or, put another way, 4 out of 5 will be missed, making this a relatively ineffective test for Down syndrome, a drawback you want to keep in mind.[69]

Many results outside of average are false positives, also one of the weaknesses of this test. In other words, the results indicate a possible birth defect when there actually is none. While higher than average levels of AFP will usually be detected in the mother's blood if her baby has a neural tube defect, a woman carrying healthy twins will also have high serum levels of AFP; a pregnancy dated further along than it really is will show lower than normal levels, falsely indicating the baby is at greater risk for Down syndrome.[70]

The follow-up process with high or low AFP levels usually involves first rechecking the age of your pregnancy and ruling out twins via ultrasound examination, and sometimes amniocentesis for further diagnosis.[71]

AFP has been replaced in some states by *multiple marker screening*. MMS is thought to be about 50 percent more accurate for women age 35 to 40, and about 70 percent more accurate for women over 40, than AFP alone.[72] If you want to avoid invasive prenatal testing, find out if multiple marker screening is available locally. (Your blood sample can be sent by overnight mail to a lab for testing if it's not.[73]) Do discuss MMS with your doctor or a genetics counselor, as its weaknesses need to be considered.

Multiple Marker Screening

MMS, also known as triple-marker screening or Expanded AFP,[74] is another prenatal test available for routine use.

MMS screens for Down syndrome, neural tube and abdominal wall defects, and trisomy 18.[75] (Trisomy 18 occurs rarely, but more often in older women. It is a severe chromosomal abnormality, usually resulting in death before the baby's first birthday,[76] if not first resulting in miscarriage.)

It is reliable between fifteen and twenty weeks, as is AFP, and the best time to have it is also at sixteen to seventeen weeks of pregnancy.[77] Although these specific weeks do give a slightly better chance of detecting a problem using multiple marker screening,[78] the real advantage (again, as with AFP testing) is in making allowances for a misdated pregnancy, along with leaving sufficient time for the option of terminating the pregnancy based on test results.

The laboratory will look for the amounts of three substances in your blood: AFP; HCG, or human chorionic gonadotropin; and UE, or unconjugated estriol.[79] When the level of AFP is higher than normal at this point in pregnancy, as mentioned earlier, the fetus may be at greater risk for NTDs and abdominal wall defects. When AFP or UE are lower than is normal, or HCG is higher, the risk of Down syndrome may be greater.[80] With MMS, you get three layers of information about your baby's health rather than just one, as with AFP.

The levels of these substances are combined with your age, along with other factors, such as your weight, week of pregnancy, and ethnic background, to give you a prediction of your *individual* risk.[81] For instance, your test results could indicate that your level of risk is the same as for a 32-year-old woman even though you are now 36, or at age 43, your risk is equivalent to that of a woman of 35. Test results are usually available within one to two weeks.[82]

Levels that fall within the range of normal are called *screen negative.* Levels that are outside the norms are called *screen positive.* As with testing for AFP alone, higher or lower than usual amounts of AFP, UE, and HCG are most often not because a birth defect exists, but because of inaccurate dating of the pregnancy, the presence of twins or triplets, or a benign variation.[83] Thus a false positive result is not infrequent. (The language is confusing; false positives are screen positive results that are *not* due to a birth defect. In other words, when a test falsely shows there might be birth defects when none actually exists.) Women with a screen positive result are offered further testing to determine whether there actually is a fetal abnormality. Two tests are generally available for follow-up at this point: an ultrasound examination and then, if needed, amniocentesis.[84]

One other weakness of this test is that the false negative rate for Down syndrome for women 35 and over is 10 to 30 percent actually exists.[85] In other words, Down syndrome that is actually present will not be detected up to almost one-third of the time. (Detection rates vary from lab to lab.[86]) For example, at age 35 MMS might miss up to 29 out of 100 Down syndrome pregnancies, and at 39, up to 13 out of 100 might miss detection.[87]

The predictive value of MMS increases with age, and thus this test is more useful for us at midlife than it is for younger women. Yet you can see that it does not approach the better than 99 percent rate of accuracy you get with amniocentesis or CVS. Although an accurate modified, personalized rate of risk is undeniably useful, for a woman uncomfortable with anything less than that near 100 percent rate, the possibility of a false negative MMS test result needs to be factored in.

Some women who are ambivalent about amniocentesis look to their MMS results to help them decide to decline it or not. More than a few midlife women do in fact choose to forgo amniocentesis. In a survey of 636 screen positive women age 35-plus, 344 of them—54 percent—chose not to have an amniocentesis.[88] In another study, although the numbers of screen positive midlife subjects was smaller, (98 women) nearly 60 percent decided against amniocentesis.[89] The authors suggested that even though these women tested positive, their decision was prompted by the fact that the percent of individual risk based on their multiple marker screening was actually lower than their generic age group risk.

Although it is important to keep the false negative rate in mind—meaning that MMS will not detect every Down syndrome pregnancy—most often this test provides accurate results for midlife women. New tests should continue to improve the detection rate. One promising one on the horizon, called *quadruple testing*, measures the level of a fourth substance found in the mother's blood called *Inhibin A* in addition to the three already tested in MMS. While data is still being collected and validated, quadruple testing may be available in some facilities in the next year or two.[90] Meanwhile, there is one more noninvasive test routinely available—ultrasound.

Ultrasound

One use of ultrasound is to help assess abnormal results from either AFP or MMS screening. Ultrasound can help in correctly dating a pregnancy, can show whether you are pregnant with twins, and often can show if a neural tube defect is present. Many abnormal AFP and MMS test results are explained with a subsequent ultrasound examination.[91]

Ultrasound works for prenatal uses by creating an image when high frequency sound waves are bounced off the fetus.[92] Still pictures can be taken at any time. A hand-held *transducer* is used either on your belly, or, for a vaginal ultrasound, a probe-shaped transducer is covered with a condom and then inserted a short way into your vagina.

Ultrasound can show a heartbeat as early as six weeks into pregnancy. Many physicians use ultrasound primarily on an as-needed basis, perhaps to confirm the age of the pregnancy as well as to look into any question about the viability of the fetus, for instance if a patient has noticed some bleeding or spotting. However, around the twelve-week mark, the baby's heartbeat can usually be heard with a *Doppler,* a small ultrasound type of device that translates motion into sound.[93] The use of a Doppler may then become routine at every visit. You should have a sonogram (another name for ultrasound) before and during any prenatal diagnostic procedure.

Your routine prenatal care may include a high-resolution, complete sonogram at eighteen weeks of pregnancy or later.[94] The anatomy of the fetus is then explored overall, in detail. Pictures taken of the baby in utero will be studied by a physician for fetal characteristics that may be associated with chromosomal abnormalities, for neural tube disorders—checked for visually at this time even with a normal alpha fetoprotein result from either AFP or MMS screening—or for any visible major malformations.

This far into pregnancy, with this much fetal development in place and evident, a trained, skilled eye can be very valuable in picking up existing or potential problems. Also, since the sex of the baby can usually be identified by mid-trimester, if it is not known through previous tests, this can certainly be a good time to find out if you wish.

Genetic counseling or a short classroom course on genetics should be offered to any woman having a baby at 35-plus. These services are sometimes included as part of prenatal care given women at midlife, in either an individual or a group setting. Taking advantage of these services can be enormously helpful in understanding the prenatal testing options available and making the choices that are right for you.

FOUR

Fertility Treatment: When, Who, and What

The majority of women age 35 to 44 *are* fertile according to a number of sources, including a national survey on fertility by the United States Department of Health and Human Services.[1] Other authoritative experts believe fertility varies by increments in the early forties, and that most women up to age 42 can have babies using their own eggs.[2] Then over 42 years, *many* but perhaps no longer most are fertile, with pregnancy being relatively rare beyond ages 44 to 45,[3] as we become increasing subfertile, and then finally infertile with menopause occurring on average at 51 years.[4]

However, governmental data shows infertility not to be on the rise among midlife women, nor, for that matter, women of any age.[5] The misconception that it is probably has to do with the fact that there simply are now greater numbers of women in their midlife years (baby boomers), coupled with the increase in availability and use of infertility services overall, not just among 35-plus women.[6] *More women* does not mean *more infertility*.

However, the chances of ending up unable to have a biological child are clearly higher over 35 and more so over 40. Therefore, whether or not you believe you would seek medical help if you don't get pregnant as quickly as you expect and hope to, as a midlife woman who wants a baby, you'll want to know *when* it is time to look into fertility treatment, *who* to turn to, and *what* to expect.

When to Consider Working with a Specialist

The overall rates of conception look something like this: 50 percent within three months, 75 percent within six months, and 95 percent within twelve months,[7] with infertility defined as not conceiving after one full year of regular, unprotected intercourse.[8] However, many women not pregnant after twelve months of giving it a full effort are actually *sub*fertile, and it may just take longer for them to conceive.[9] An infertile woman technically has *no* chance of conceiving. Subfertile women have at least some chance of conceiving, especially with the advances in reproductive medicine in recent years.[10]

Women under 35 who have not conceived within a year should discuss their situation with their ob/gyn. At midlife, however, the biological clock comes into play. When your chances of conceiving are time-limited, you don't want too much time to slip by without taking maximum advantage of your present degree of fertility.

Thus, within the field of fertility medicine, waiting no longer than a period of six months without conceiving is recommended for women over 35;[11] for women 39 and over, some infertility experts suggest that if not pregnant after three months, they may want to seriously consider getting medical help.[12] Keep in mind that not conceiving after three months or six months does not necessarily mean anything is reproductively wrong, the same way it would not have when you were younger. However, more often than for a younger woman, even a period of months can be critical.

In fact, some physicians advise any woman over 39 to go directly to an infertility specialist rather than a regular ob/gyn for a basic reproductive work-up.[13] Further, women in these following groups are *strongly* advised to consider consulting immediately with a specialist: (1) if you are 39 and over and have never conceived, as you do not then have "proven fertility"; (2) if you are 42 or over; or (3) if you have previously found out that your FSH and E2 levels are marginal or high.[14]

The three- and six-month time guides pose a dilemma of sorts for women in their middle years. Although many older women conceive as quickly as the average 25-year-old, it generally takes longer. Chances are that getting pregnant at midlife is more a matter of time. Yet, as more and more time passes, we come closer to the end of our fertile years. So do you give it more time and let nature utterly take its course? Some women and their partners feel very strongly about this and are comfortable enough with time limits on fertility to be relaxed in waiting beyond physician guidelines. Or is it wiser to act on the possibility that your own fertility endpoint may in fact be way too close for comfort?

There is no right or wrong turn here, philosophically speaking. Whichever way you believe you would lean if you do come to this juncture will most likely be the best fit for you. However, if you are certain you would never turn to fertility medicine, you might find it interesting to know that it ranges from very noninvasive assessments to very thorough reproductive evaluations, and from minor noninvasive treatment to quite involved, assisted reproductive technologies.

Some couples find it terribly useful just to have their problem diagnosed, along with some straightforward advice about how to best proceed toward having a baby given their situation. Next steps are often much more obvious when all the cards are on the table rather than when you are dealing with big unknowns.

Working with a good specialist to take advantage of the full range of options available for diagnosis and treatment of fertility problems is reassuring and heartening for many women. Yet even being certain that you would want to see a specialist may not put an end to the mixed feelings you may have about turning to fertility medicine.

Despite the hopeful or determined feelings you carry with you into that first consultation, the two of you might also feel that turning to outside help is discomfiting and disappointing, even violating. It's not easy to accept that getting pregnant is something you may not be able to make happen totally on your own. It may also be all too easy to imagine that in turning to fertility medicine, even if only for a consultation, you are taking the first step in finding out you are infertile.

Some women also keenly feel a sense of loss in that the naturalness of simply making a baby together with their husband has been thwarted. That naturalness may even feel violated, depending on the kind of treatment your doctor suggests. The feeling is temporary for most women, however, fading away once you are pregnant or at least after the baby is born, when you and your husband are now mother and father, together.

Choosing a Fertility Specialist

Your surest choice as a midlife woman looking for a fertility specialist, and especially if you are 39 or older, is a *reproductive endocrinologist*. This specialist is a gynecologist who studies how hormones interact with the reproductive system and how reproductive hormones interact with other systems in the body. However, not all REs are mainly trained in or concentrate their practices on treating infertility.[15]

Screening and interviewing will give you the best shot at ending up with the right specialist for you. (A list of the questions to ask to help you in choosing a fertility specialist follows this discussion.) In the process of your initial telephone screening, you will want to ask if the physician primarily works with fertility patients. Secondly, you want to know if he or she is board certified. A board certified RE will have successfully completed a fellowship in reproductive endocrinology, along with advanced comprehensive testing in this specific field of medicine. Also asking if the specialist has done a fellowship in your initial phone call.[16]

You'll also want a reproductive endocrinologist who can offer you the full range of fertility services, from the simplest to the most advanced reproductive technologies.[17] Not all of them are trained in advanced procedures, or stay on top of new ones as they emerge.

Chances are you won't need advanced procedures, nor is every couple interested in going through a procedure like in vitro fertilization (more to come on this type of treatment). However, when you have the advantage of the whole array of fertility measures as options, you have a greater possibility of receiving both the most effective treatment and the one you are most comfortable with.

A physician uncomfortable with your questions, or one whose answers are not easily forthcoming or seem evasive, should make you think twice. Beyond the credentials and professional presentation, keep in mind two other factors.

First, does the specialist have expertise with fertility patients over 35? He or she needs to consider your age along with your reproductive condition. For example, the step-wise progression that typically characterizes fertility treatment, beginning with the simplest forms before the patient tries the more involved ones, will probably not be the best choice for an older woman with few months to waste because of a marginal FSH or E2 levels.[18]

Second, if you are close to or over 40, does he or she have expertise with fertility patients in the over 40 group? Does the specialist have a positive attitude about working with 40-plus women and their partners? Not all of them do. Some specialists are reluctant to treat women 40 and over based on an image factor; their rates of success are higher with younger women. Others will draw the line at some treatments, in effect doing a halfhearted job, limiting your options to lower-level protocols such as many cycles of fertility drugs or repeated intrauterine inseminations. If he or she does not include the most advanced treatments as a possibility for you in your initial consultation, it may be that you are being written off because of your age.[19]

You should know about the *rule of four*.[20] Low-level treatments such as medication and intrauterine insemination should be repeated no more than four times each. Of course, there are pregnancies that have come from subsequent cycles, but it's useful to go in knowing the general rule.

QUESTIONS TO ASK ON THE PHONE

1. Are you a reproductive endocrinologist?

2. Do you work primarily with fertility patients?

3. Did you complete a fellowship in reproductive endocrinology?

4. Are you board certified in reproductive endocrinology?

5. Do you have expertise with women over 35? What percentage of your patients are over 35? What are your feelings about working with patients in this age group? (Listen for what he or she actually says as well as for what you hear between the lines.)

6. For 40-plus women: Do you have expertise with women over 40? What percentage of your patients are over 40? What are your feelings about working with patients in this age group? (Listen for both the spoken answer and between the lines.)

7. What is the range of fertility treatments you offer: Hormonal therapy? Intrauterine insemination (IUI)? In vitro insemination (IVF)? Gamete intrafallopian transfer (GIFT)? Zygote intrafallopian transfer (ZIFT)? IVF or ZIFT with donor eggs?

*   *   *

Here are some additional points to be on the alert for in an interview setting to help you assess whether you might be in good hands with this physician:[21]

1. The initial consultation takes from sixty to ninety minutes.

2. The tests and examinations involved in the basic work-up are specified.

3. The basic work-up is planned for completion in one or two cycles (months).

4. The basic work-up is to be implemented immediately.

5. A range of treatment options is presented.

6. The advantages and disadvantages of each option are explained.

7. Treatment with the most expensive procedures are not promoted as either the first or your only chance for becoming pregnant unless there is supporting evidence.

8. The costs involved are clearly discussed. Specialized care can be very expensive; you want to know how much it will cost.

Choosing an Ob/gyn for Fertility Care

When working with a reproductive endocrinologist is not an option—because of access, self-determined treatment limits, financial or other considerations—another possibility is working with your ob/gyn. Many ob/gyns, although not board certified in reproductive medicine, have a special interest in the field of infertility and have spent many years diagnosing causes and treating fertility patients competently and well.

While working with a RE should offer patients an efficiency in their treatment that comes with advanced study, along with day-in and day-out experience—an advantage to seriously consider at midlife—certainly not every certified fertility specialist will know more or do a better job than a general ob/gyn who is truly knowledgeable and experienced at treating fertility problems. There most certainly are midlife women who do go on to have their babies after receiving fertility treatment from their regular gynecologist.

The potential drawbacks lie in the areas of diagnosis and treatment. For instance, the higher-tech procedures, such as in vitro fertilization, are typically not part of their standard repertoire, and FSH and E2 testing may not be routine. Yet an ob/gyn can usually do most if not all of the tests that might be involved in the basic work-up,[22] and some women and their partners are reluctant to take the next steps with a reproductive endocrinologist even when time is an issue.

It's a very important and very individual choice, another one to think about or talk through. Give yourself time to thoroughly weigh all the different pieces involved to make the decision you are most comfortable with.

The Basic Work-up

It will be to your advantage to walk into your physician interview knowing what to expect. First, there should be a discussion of your menstrual, reproductive, and coital history. You'll be asked about previous pregnancies, how long you've been trying to conceive, how frequently you have intercourse.[23] You'll feel more comfortable if you are already familiar with the more common fertility tests that will be discussed as part of your basic work-up. Below is an outline of the names of each, along with a brief description.

1. *Semen analysis.* This can be done anytime. About 45 percent of infertility is related to a "male factor."[24] Some days of abstaining from ejaculation are required (three days is typical). A sample of your husband's sperm is collected by masturbation either at home or in the doctor's office. The sample is checked for sperm count, motility, and formation.[25]

2. *Postcoital test.* This test is performed mid-cycle, just before ovulation. Several hours after intercourse, you will go to your doctor's office to have a sample of your cervical mucus evaluated. With your feet in stirrups while on an examining table, your doctor will insert a speculum and take a sample.[26] Known also as Huhner's Test,[27] it evaluates sperm survival in your cervical mucus after intercourse.

3. *Hysterosalpingogram, or HSG.* This test is done around day seven of your cycle.[28] With your feet in stirrups while on the exam table, a small tube is placed in your cervix.[29] Your cervix is dilated if the tube cannot be placed without doing so.[30] A special dye is injected through the tube, which flows into your uterus. The dye makes blockages in your Fallopian tubes or uterine abnormalities visible on a TV screen with the use of an X-ray machine.[31]

4. *Laparoscopy.* Performed in the first half of the cycle. During this surgical procedure, a tiny scope is passed through a small incision made in your navel.[32] The physician can make a more thorough anatomical assessment by directly viewing the uterus, ovaries, and tubes for adhesions and endometriosis, for example.

5. *Hysteroscopy.* This may be done at the same time as a laparoscopy. A special scope is guided through the vagina and into the uterus for a direct examination of the tissue and anatomy.[33]

6. *Hormonal tests. FSH* and *E2* are tested on the third day of your cycle via a blood test to check for egg quality.[34]

Prolactin, a pituitary hormone, is tested in your blood anytime. High levels can inhibit ovulation or the quality of ovulation.[35]

An *endometrial biopsy* is performed one to three days before your period. On the exam table with your feet in stirrups, a small instrument with a sharp top will be carefully inserted through your dilated cervix. A tiny piece of the tissue lining the uterus— the endometrium—is removed.[36] Your doctor will look at the thickness of the endometrium to determine whether enough progesterone has been produced. A certain level of progesterone is necessary for the fertilized egg to implant and grow in the early part of pregnancy.[37]

Not all these tests may be part of your physician's basic evaluation. The basic work-up varies from physician to physician, as well as from patient to patient.

Assisted Reproductive Technologies

Although relatively few women of any age in fertility treatment actually use the high-tech assisted reproductive technologies, or ARTs,[38] I'm including them here because one or more of these procedures is likely to be recommended to an 35-plus woman in fertility treatment. There are certainly middle-of-the-road levels of treatment that are appropriate for midlife women depending on their individual fertility profile—hormonal medications and restorative surgery, for example—but you'll want to be aware of these most advanced ones if you are looking for a specialist who offers the full range of fertility care. They should be discussed as options in your initial consultation. The following will give you basic information about five of the collection of procedures known mostly by their initials.

INTRAUTERINE INSEMINATION

Intrauterine Insemination, or IUI, is also called artificial insemination. (AIH stands for artificial insemination husband, AID for artificial insemination donor.) This is actually a low-tech procedure,[39] but is the most common of all the ARTs.[40] Sperm is placed into the uterus with the use of a catheter, close to the opening of one of your Fallopian tubes,[41] where an egg will be released from your ovary and fertilized.

IN VITRO FERTILIZATION

In vitro fertilization, or IVF, is the most common of the advanced procedures.[42] Egg and sperm are placed together in a laboratory plate. (This is where the "test tube baby" description comes from.) When the eggs are fertilized, the embryos are carefully moved to the uterus to implant and develop.[43]

GAMETE INTRAFALLOPIAN TRANSFER

In gamete intrafallopian transfer, or GIFT, eggs and sperm are placed into a Fallopian tube via a small incision made in the area of one or both tubes.[44] Once an egg is fertilized, it travels as it normally would through the tube and into the uterus.

ZYGOTE INTRAFALLOPIAN TRANSFER

Zygote intrafallopian transfer, or ZIFT, borrows from IVF and GIFT.[45] Your eggs are fertilized in a laboratory dish before being placed in the Fallopian tube to float to the uterus and implant.

DONOR EGGS

When conceiving with your own eggs is no longer a possibility, pregnancy with your partner's sperm and a donor's egg is one option, and midlife women in fertility care are most likely to have this alternative presented to them than are younger patients. The crux of this process involves fertilization of the donor's egg in the lab with the father's sperm. The viable embryos are then transferred into the recipient's uterus as with IVF, or to a Fallopian tube, as in ZIFT.[46]

Think twice about choosing a physician who recommends egg donation as your only chance for becoming pregnant *solely* based on your age; the physician's bias is showing if this is the case. Age is obviously a factor that affects the quality of the eggs, but experts do not consider it the best single indicator of your chances. FSH and E2 levels are thought to be better predictors.[47]

If you find yourself considering fertility treatment, you may want to know more about the details involved in the whole process, along with the nuts and bolts of practical issues such as insurance and costs. *How to Be a Successful Fertility Patient*, by Peggy Robin, is a thorough and readable resource.[48]

FIVE

Embracing Pregnancy Again

Here you are, looking to have a baby at midlife. Chances are, you're more than willing to make the enormous changes that are called for when a baby comes into your life. Most of us in our midlife years do well in negotiating our way through the world of baby-child-parenting, one that is often hugely new and different from the kind of life experiences we've mastered thus far.

With so much else in life already settled—relationship, career, self-exploration, travel—we're usually very clear about how much a child matters to us. Any quaking in confidence is overshadowed by the longing for a child of our own. All of which adds up to the simple fact that you are ready to become a mother.

The readiness that you feel can't and shouldn't be tempered; the desire to be pregnant, to have a baby, to create a family with children, runs deep. However, there is one pregnancy experience that no one is really ready for—miscarriage.

Miscarriage

The overall rate of miscarriage, 20 percent,[1] comes as something of a surprise to many women. Most of us don't grow up with a point of view encompassing pregnancy loss as a real possibility, or as a normal although undeniably difficult, part of the total pregnancy experience. Yet even higher numbers are sometimes quoted, to account for lost *subclinical pregnancies*. Some professionals believe that many pregnancies begin and end almost as soon as they start; often before a standard pregnancy test is taken, (usually done around ten to fourteen days after ovulation), and before the physical signs of pregnancy become apparent. When miscarriage happens this early, your period might be just a few days or a week late or may even start right on time without any delay at all caused by conceiving.[2]

The overall 2 out of 10 figure reflects the frequency of pregnancy loss for women of all ages taken together as a group. The numbers start low, at 9.5 percent for 20 to 24-year-olds, increasing only slightly through age 34. They hop up to approximately 18 percent at 35 to 39 years and then, to about 34 percent at 40 to 44 years.[3]

Despite the increases, these percentages mean that *most* women over 35 and over 40 *never* have a brush with pregnancy loss. With a positive pregnancy test most of us do go on to have babies. In your middle to late thirties, your chances for carrying to term are better than 82 percent, meaning even fewer miscarriages than the overall rate; after 40, they are around 66 percent, still good. The odds are in your favor; it just takes a little more patience . . . and a little more luck.

Why more luck? The one word answer is *chromosomes*. Chromosomal abnormalities are responsible for 50 percent or more of all miscarriages.[4] They are both the major cause of miscarriage in the first trimester and the only definite, universally agreed upon cause of these early pregnancy losses.[5] That older women have more eggs that are not chromosomally perfect explains at least in part why they have more miscarriages.

There is an element of simply waiting for a good egg in midlife pregnancy. It *is* more a matter of chance for us than it is for a younger woman that a perfect one will be ovulated each month; and the chances are excellent to good, depending on where you are in the midlife years, that it will, if not every month, then often enough for you to successfully conceive and carry to term.

Outside of chromosomal abnormalities, a long list of conditions are considered *possible* causes of miscarriage. Successfully diagnosing the reason for a miscarriage can be frustrating, as even an experienced clinician who makes full use of medical tests will find the same suspicious condition to be the problem for one woman, but not for another.

What follows, therefore, is a short list of causes that may more often affect a woman at 35-plus trying to have a baby. Despite the lack of certainty for any cause but chromosomal abnormalities, it's a good idea to have at least a basic understanding of what these are.

Much of the following is drawn from material in the book *Motherhood After Miscarriage* by Dr. Kathleen Diamond. This book is a wonderful resource for a reader wanting to take a more thorough look at the subject of pregnancy loss.[6]

CAUSES

Luteal Phase Deficiency

The second half of a woman's cycle is called the *luteal phase*. The word *deficiency* refers to the inadequate production of the hormone progesterone. If enough progesterone is not present at this juncture, the endometrium, the lining of the uterus, will not thicken and become rich with nourishing substances needed to support the embryo during the first weeks of pregnancy.[7] LPD may therefore be suspected when miscarriage occurs before 8 weeks.[8]

The eggs in the ovaries each nest in a collection of cells that form a "follicle." When an egg is released for ovulation, the empty follicle becomes what is called the *corpus luteum*, which produces the progesterone crucial to the embryo's survival.

A number of possibilities explain insufficient amounts of progesterone. One in particular—not universally accepted, but logical—may be more applicable for women in their middle years than for younger women. This theory suggests that the inadequacy of progesterone in the luteal phase can be traced to the quality of a woman's follicles, which, like older eggs, also decreases over the years.[9]

LPD can be chronic or intermittent. An occasional imperfect cycle may be commonplace for all women, part of the package of being human rather than a reproductive machine. In fact, many women have cycles where not enough progesterone is present and yet have no problems conceiving and carrying to term.[10]

Chronic LPD means progesterone deficiencies in many or most cycles. Because of the effects of age on the follicles, a single early pregnancy loss at 35-plus might be explained by LPD; with recurrent miscarriages prior to eight weeks, a chronic condition becomes a prime suspect.

Fortunately, not only will few of us experience repeated miscarriages, but LPD is easy to treat. Many physicians prescribe progesterone suppositories (or sometimes injections) for women who clearly have luteal phase deficiencies.[11] Some prescribe them even when LPD is merely considered a reasonable possibility, to cover all the bases.[12] The natural form of progesterone usually prescribed is not thought to have harmful side effects (unlike the synthetic form) even if a sufficient level of progesterone is being produced by your body.[13]

Uterine Abnormalities

Structural uterine abnormalities are infrequent.[14] Yet, although relatively rare, they are more often found in DES daughters (see Chapter One, page 17) many of whom are now in their midlife years.

A "T-shaped" uterus is more common among women whose mothers took DES while pregnant.[15] Theoretically, this anatomical configuration reduces the surface area available for an embryo to implant, and may interfere with the circulation of hormones necessary to the embryo's growth. Although it cannot be treated surgically, hormone treatments may be used to help a woman avoid a pregnancy loss.[16] It is thought to contribute to the occurrence of a miscarriage rather than being the primary cause.

The second uterine problem more common for DES daughters is called *incompetent cervix*, which is a cervix that dilates way too early rather than remaining tightly closed as it should until about the time the baby is due. An incompetent cervix may be responsible when a late miscarriage occurs, meaning one beyond the first trimester. To treat this condition, the cervix is sewn closed in a procedure called *cerclage*, (pronounced *sirclawj*), with the stitches generally remaining in place until they are removed a few weeks before the baby is expected, at about 37 weeks.[17]

NON-CAUSES

Fortunately, there is much less ambiguity about what does not jeopardize a pregnancy than about causes other than genetic abnormalities. For instance, it is not believed that using a computer or microwave,[18] or exercise or intercourse,[19] all common concerns when it comes to pregnancy loss, will make you more likely to miscarry.

Limiting or avoiding intercourse is advised shortly before birth and when a current pregnancy is treated as a high-risk one because of problems in the past, such as a premature delivery. Most couples are otherwise counseled to have comfort be their guide.[20] There are standard guidelines for exercising, the details of which are covered in Chapter Six.

Fears that working with a computer will cause a miscarriage are not well founded. Two studies done in the 1980s did not find a direct link between computer use and pregnancy loss, but suggested there might be a connection between miscarriage and a woman's level of activity.

One study of several thousand women found no difference in the number of miscarriages for workers who used computers and those who didn't, but were equally inactive. Another did find an increase for women sitting at computers over twenty hours per week, but similarly concluded that other factors, such as inactivity, were the real problem.[21]

Microwaves have not been studied specifically regarding miscarriage, yet it is doubtful that using one could trigger a pregnancy loss, or birth defects, for that matter. Microwaves use electromagnetic waves that dissipate over short distances. These waves generate heat rather than work in any way to change the composition of cells and create mutations as can happen with exposure to the kind of radiation used with X-rays.[22] Most microwaves have safety features that automatically shut the oven down if there are leaks. Should such a safety mechanism fail, you can rest assured that by taking a few steps away from the oven after you turn it on, you'll be effectively out of range of the electromagnetic waves it generates in seconds.

TESTING

More and more physicians are now testing to determine the cause of a miscarriage after at most two first trimester pregnancy losses in a row, and after one in the second trimester.[23] However, beyond the cost factor, there are several reasons some physicians still will not test until after the old standard guideline of three in a row.

Chromosomal abnormalities are believed to be the cause of most single miscarriages. The usefulness of testing then comes into question, as a chromosomal problem is neither treatable nor preventable, nor expected to be repeated in the next pregnancy. Along this same line is the belief that outside of chromosomes most conditions that contribute to pregnancy loss are temporary— intermittent LPD, for example—and will self-cure without any medical intervention.

So, from a strictly medical point of view, a first miscarriage is by and large viewed as a normal part of reproduction, more a matter of bad luck than a sign of an enduring problem that would prevent a successful pregnancy the next time a woman conceives.

If a second (or third) miscarriage occurs in the midlife years, it is about as likely to be caused by chromosomes as a first.[24] (Chromosomal abnormalities are at the root of a second and third pregnancy loss less often for younger women).[25] At the same time other treatable problems (LPD is one) also become more of a factor.

Hence, diagnosing and treating a condition responsible for an unsuccessful pregnancy after two miscarriages, even after one, makes good sense for middle-years women, especially those in their late thirties and early forties. Why? Because the limits on a midlife woman's fertility mean it's essential to use the time she has well. The time it takes to conceive, miscarry, recover (both physically and psychologically) three times before testing begins adds up to many wasted months. The emotional costs of another miscarriage, along with the fears a second one further creates about being able to have a baby, also need to be considered.

Testing after one or two miscarriages gives a woman a quicker answer to the heart-wrenching question, "Is there something wrong with me?" Usually, the answer is no. While it's impossible to totally shake the uncertainty a miscarriage engenders the next time you're pregnant, this information can be an enormous relief, in and of itself an important reason to be tested early.

Your Subsequent Pregnancy

The forces of biology happen to work in our favor when it comes to having children. Given a good egg, a good sperm, and well-timed intercourse, the basic movement of life supports the creation of a baby. Life is simply geared toward reproduction and survival at a biological level. For example, until a plant dies because of disease or perhaps lack of water or light, it simply never stops growing. A pregnancy is like that, most often ending only when something is very wrong.

In fact, most of us who have a miscarriage will go on to have a baby. Further, as devastating as a pregnancy loss can be, it does confirm that you can conceive and that your reproductive system is basically working the way it should. One miscarriage rarely indicates the following pregnancy will be lost, and the vast majority of women will be successful the very next time they are pregnant.[26]

REASSURING SIGNS

A pregnancy subsequent to a miscarriage does not necessarily mean instant feelings of pure joy or the free flow of maternal fantasies. Usually it brings a mixture of feelings: You're happy to be pregnant, but almost afraid to feel hopeful that you will be able to have a baby this time around. Fears of another loss can vary from mild to tremendous. How a woman responds to her subsequent pregnancy is a very individual matter, with no one place along this continuum more normal or fitting than any other.

Some women need just a little "evidence" to regain enough confidence in their bodies to feel comfortable in their new pregnancy. During the earlier weeks when fears run the strongest, there are several encouraging signs to look for, beginning of course, with conceiving again.

Those first signs that you're pregnant again are greatly reassuring to most women. A missed period, breast tenderness, and fatigue are some typical early clues. There's a feeling of relief, as the question "Can I conceive again?" has been answered. And now you have another chance to have a child.

After you conceive, the hormone HCG (human chorionic gonadotropin) will go up and up. While the range of normal is very broad, in your earliest weeks it will double about every forty-eight hours as your pregnancy progresses. The rate of increase will begin to slow down once the HCG reaches a certain level.[27] Then around your tenth week, the total amount of HCG produced peaks and begins to taper off.[28]

Your doctor may have the HCG levels in your blood checked if there's a question about the safety of your pregnancy. When doubts arise—for instance, if you are spotting or your symptoms seem to have waned and you just don't feel as pregnant as you were—you will be encouraged by these steadily increasing numbers.

For many women, viewing the baby's heart beating on an ultrasound monitor brings it home that something really is going on in there! Visible on ultrasound as early as your sixth week, that tiny pulsing spot, seen with your own eyes, is reassuring, to say the least; it is absolutely thrilling and deeply moving to catch this first glimpse of the baby. You won't be able to take your eyes from the screen!

The ultrasound equipment that allows you to see a baby in the womb can also be used to measure it. When adequate growth is documented around eight weeks of pregnancy, with a heartbeat also visible, you have another positive piece of evidence.[29] These tiny measurements give you an idea of whether the baby's size at that point is within the range of normal.

Reaching your ten-week mark, with movement now visible on ultrasound along with a heartbeat, is further cause for reassurance that your pregnancy appears to be going well.[30] The baby is now out of the embryo stage and officially called a *fetus*.

These reassuring signs are listed below for quick referral:

1. Conceiving again.

2. Your level of HCG doubles about every forty-eight hours in your earliest weeks of pregnancy.

3. Seeing a tiny heartbeat on ultrasound examination, as early as six weeks.

4. Documented, adequate growth, plus a heartbeat, at eight weeks, both registered through ultrasound.

5. Reaching ten weeks, plus fetal movement along with a heartbeat, on ultrasound.

These are all hallmarks that begin to add up to a viable pregnancy. In fact, when a fetal heartbeat and movement are visible through ultrasound around the end of the first trimester, the possibility of a miscarriage becomes very low, between 2 percent and 5 percent.[31] Thus, the chances of carrying to term are then as high as 98 percent. Although the possibility of pregnancy loss after this point may be higher at midlife than it is for younger women[32] passing through this period with a pregnancy intact, while not a guarantee, is a good sign.

Stages and Strategies

STAGE ONE—WAIT AND SEE

Many women, however, do not rebound quickly from a miscarriage. While the evidence that your current pregnancy appears to be secure is a most welcome relief, the earlier pregnancy loss deals an enduring blow. A woman with this experience may spend most of the early months (or more!) figuratively holding her breath regarding the fate of her pregnancy.

While you are indeed happy to be pregnant again, this time you're also likely to take a more measured approach to it all. You'll probably find yourself being not only extra judicious in whom you chose to share the news with, but also more reserved in your own excitement. There's a sense of stepping back from your own feelings that wasn't there the first time you were pregnant. It's a time of "wait and see," and is the first of three stages many women experience in their subsequent pregnancy.

(If you regained your sense of equilibrium relatively soon after your miscarriage, you may not find this section particularly relevant. You may want to skip ahead to the last section of this chapter, titled "The Positive Reality)."

STAGE TWO—APPREHENSION AND UNCERTAINTY

The next stage begins when your worries about another miscarriage become strong and pervasive. You may feel as though your apprehension leaves no moment untouched for a while.

A first miscarriage is often a completely unexpected shock. The belief that conception and pregnancy are one seamless event is turned on its head as the sequence of one event, pregnancy, followed by the next, having a baby, is disrupted. Your sense of order flies out the window; you're left unsure about what to expect now. The uncertainty spills over into other areas of your life, and is part of why overall feelings of vulnerability and insecurity can be part of the aftermath of a miscarriage.

Guilt and Self-Blame

Sometimes mixed into the pot is a sense of guilt for not trying to have a baby sooner. You may blame yourself for being in your present situation. You may be angry with yourself for not realizing that pregnancy could be a more complicated project in your middle years than earlier.

Yet your self-criticism and guilt don't change the fact that most women have no problems with their midlife pregnancies. It could have easily been an effortless and smooth process for you too. Because miscarriage is not uncommon at any age, you will never know for certain if yours was age-related or not. You may have wanted equally as much as a child to be in a stable relationship that didn't come along until later, or to be otherwise secure with a number of issues settled in your life (such as developing a career or resolving parent/child dynamics you didn't want to come into play with your own children).

You may not even have known until close to your mid-thirties or your forties how much you wanted a baby. Even if you were acutely aware that midlife was not a biologically optimal time to try to get pregnant, try to hold on to this thought: Whether or not you made your earlier choice consciously, chances are you took

the totality of your life circumstances—inner as well as outer—
into consideration. Whether you did so purposely and piece by
piece, or more from an impression of your life as a whole, the
odds are good that it was the right one at the time.

Strategies

Before we go onto the last stage, let's turn to three strategies
that can help you more easily pass through these first two.

BE YOUR OWN BEST ADVOCATE

First, you need to know that your feelings are natural. It will
take a while for you to trust that nature's course can be positive,
meaning that you will be able to carry to term or close enough to
have a healthy baby. When enough time has passed and all is
going well, you will feel much more relaxed in your pregnancy.
While you may not be able to specify or even anticipate that point
until it actually arrives, it *will* come. Until then, you can help
yourself by educating yourself.

Your best source of information about your own pregnancy is
the physician or other medical professional involved in your prenatal care. Ask questions about your concerns. Don't hesitate to
call or set up extra appointments to discuss what's on your mind
for fear of being a bother. Be thorough. The more information you
have about your pregnancy, the more solid you will feel in it.

Has something occurred or does something seem to be missing in
your body experience that makes you uneasy? For instance, has your
nausea lessened or ceased entirely? Although it does at some point for
almost all women, you might nevertheless feel some concern if your
nausea has thus far been a reassuring sign that you are still pregnant.

Breast tenderness and fullness can noticeably fluctuate even in
the first few months when breast changes are dramatic. Does it
concern you that they appear to be less full or are not as sensitive
to the touch as they once were? Or are you experiencing uterine
twinges that feel something like the ones you had before, and fear
they are the beginning of the end?

None of these examples necessarily signals a pending miscarriage. As your pregnancy continues, you will begin to discover what is normal for you in this particular pregnancy, and when it feels like something is wrong. But for now, getting information about your body experience will help set your mind at ease.

TEN STRATEGIES FOR DEALING WITH FEAR

You also want to make an extra effort to be self-caring and to find sources of emotional sustenance. The payoff for doing so can be enormously helpful. Support from your husband, family, and friends and the care and nurturing you give yourself will bolster your strength and resilience; you will probably discover a tenacity you may not have known you had, or rediscover an inner strength you'd forgotten you could call on.

Here are some strategies for dealing with fear through self-care and nurturing.

1. *Know that you can make it through this difficult time.* Many of us have waited out uncertain pregnancies before you, and have given birth to healthy, beautiful babies. It's important to know that this is a period of time to just *get through.*

Being worried or afraid doesn't make fears come true. Nor is there shame or indignity in feeling fearful. Don't let anyone criticize you for worrying too much or for not being able to relax, for not having more faith or for being too intense. In your own time, given the evidence you need, your fear *will* diminish.

2. *Allow yourself to become absorbed in your pregnancy.* Many women find themselves wrapped up in their pregnancies, especially the first time around. Pregnancy happens in your body, the reminder is always with you, and you literally can't get away from the object of your concern. Being absorbed in your pregnancy is to be expected, and even more so if there are concerns about how it will all turn out.

3.   *Do at least one thing that matters to you every day that has nothing to do with pregnancy or babies.* Although it is natural to be absorbed in it, it's also important that you are living a life that matters to you, *now*. Don't put on hold everything else that makes life worthwhile for you until a baby comes. If not much else is meaningful to you besides having a baby, take a few moments to try the following exercise.

Set a timer for two minutes. Then begin writing one-word or short-phrase descriptions of what you find interesting in life: activities or pastimes that naturally attract your interest. These are things you don't have to talk yourself into wanting to do in any way, that you are attracted to for no other reason than you like doing them or think you would if you let yourself follow your natural inclinations.

Write without pausing so you don't have time to think your way out of listing an interest. When two minutes are up, review what you have on your sheet of paper. Choose your top five. Prioritize them, with number one being your favorite, and write them on a separate sheet in that order.

Starting with your top choice, find some way, *any way* even if just for minutes per day, to bring that interest into your life. Let yourself have it for a month. The next month, if you want to sample another interest, go on to number two. After a month of number two, go on to number three, and so on. Again, it can be very helpful during the stage of apprehension to be presently involved in something that both matters to you and has nothing to do with pregnancy.

4.   *Do at least one caring thing for yourself every day.* For example, take a bubble bath, or use a specially scented skin lotion, have a quiet cup of tea. Buy yourself a beautiful rose, write in a journal— anything that feels nurturing to body or soul. This strategy can overlap with number three, but has more to do with directly caring for your body and nurturing your inner self.

5.   *Don't read books about miscarriage unless you are very, very certain that to do so would be helpful to you at this time.* Although it is a great step forward that miscarriage is increasingly recognized as a real loss that can bring a well of sadness and grief, now is not the best time to focus on pregnancy loss. It is inevitable that reading about it will highlight the very fear you are presently taking steps to move through.

6. *Talk about your feelings.* Speak with your husband, a trusted friend, religious counselor, or professional therapist about your fears for this pregnancy. Although no one can guarantee its safety, it often helps just to express your feelings rather than keep them silently bottled up.

7. *Monitor your thoughts.* You may find it helpful to limit the amount of time during the day you allow your fears to be foremost in your mind. Most of us can exert a degree of control over our feelings, especially if we already have a safe and supportive place to air them such as described above in number six.

Monitoring your thoughts doesn't mean you shut the door on noticing signs that something could be wrong with your pregnancy, or that you cease to check with your prenatal care provider about your questions and concerns. Rather, you are making the decision to be firm with your fear, in effect saying *Enough!* to the thoughts and fantasies of what could go wrong. To do this you can employ the tactic of firmly saying to yourself, *No!*, or *Not now!*

For instance, you would say *Not now!* to your anxious feelings each time they come up in a day, except for the two fifteen-minute periods set aside to purposely let your scary feelings and thoughts run wild. Or you could save them all for thirty minutes every evening or give yourself time in the morning to sit and simply focus on your apprehensive feelings for half an hour.

Creating parameters that set time aside for these feelings, but set limits on them too can help you cope as well as make room for your good feelings about being pregnant to be a bigger part of the picture.

8. *Join a support group that specifically focuses on issues and feelings pertaining to a subsequent pregnancy.* If you can't find any such group in your area, consider starting one yourself. It can be well worth the effort to know you are not alone in your concerns about being pregnant after going through a miscarriage.

9. *Develop a plan.* Sometimes considering what you will do if this pregnancy is not successful relieves some of the stress of living with uncertainty about the outcome. Knowing that you will definitely try again or that this is the last time you are willing to go through this can restore a sense of control over your own destiny.

10. *Reserve time for relaxation exercises, prayer, or meditation.* If you have no spare time to set aside for any of these, try this as-you-go relaxation technique:

When an apprehensive thought or a wave of fear runs through you, make yourself take slow, measured breaths. Without trying to push your feelings away, shift your attention to your breath, just noticing that you are breathing in and breathing out.

After a minute or so, you may find that you feel at least a little more relaxed and can enjoy a brief respite from your anxious feelings.

Your capacity for endurance and your resiliency are now being called upon. During this time it is important, and appropriate, to take extra measures to help yourself best get through it. Try all of these or start with the one or two you like the most. And keep in mind that at some point, your feelings of apprehension and uncertainty will lessen and give way, as you enter the next stage.

STAGE THREE—MAKING PEACE WITH FEAR

As time passes by and you're still pregnant, a measure of faith and confidence in your capacity to have a baby will return. If your miscarriage ended early in your first trimester, your turning point may arrive when you pass the week of pregnancy at which it happened. Or you may only begin to relax when you start into your second trimester still pregnant. For some this shift takes place much, much later, even at a point they can't even predict. Rather, one day they simply feel ready to embrace being pregnant again. You are in the third stage when you finally feel free to be excited about having a baby.

The faith you feel now is not the unquestioned sort you might have had at the very beginning in the inevitable progression of pregnancy to birth. That kind of innocence, that level of comfort, is gone forever. This is knowledge born from actual experience.

You may still hold your breath until the baby is born, but you're also now breathing a lot easier. While you probably won't ever take the security of your pregnancy for granted, a level of confidence in its safety will continue to grow. And as you begin to celebrate your pregnancy, you'll start letting back in the wonderful fantasies you earlier put away. Now you can start to cheer the fact that you are not only a pregnant woman, but also a mother to be.

The Positive Reality

Miscarriage is more of a concern in midlife pregnancy. Does this mean as a woman over 35 you should go into the process of having a baby *expecting* to have a miscarriage? No—but neither would it be a total anomaly for any of us, especially as we move into our late thirties and forties. While it is not accurate to say the chances are good that you will lose a pregnancy, it is apt to say the chances are real. Taking this to heart as a midlife woman hoping to have a baby can help you maintain a feeling of balance and sense of perspective that will support you in the long run. Just as important to keep in mind, however, is this: The fact that miscarriage is a greater possibility when we're older does not change the fact that, as a group, *we are much more likely to have a baby than we are to have a miscarriage.*

II

BEING PREGNANT

SIX

Pregnancy Month by Month

The stand-out issues of midlife pregnancy—fertility limits ("old eggs"), miscarriage, prenatal diagnosis, and age-related infertility—are important ones to be aware of when getting ready to have a baby in your midlife years. However, being pregnant over 35 and at 40-plus is also, "just being pregnant."

And, "just being pregnant" is an incomparable experience. The enormous number of bodily processes at work, the physical metamorphosis that unfolds in front of your eyes, even week by week, the depth and intensity of your emotions throughout, all topped off by the fact that a baby—*your* baby—is actually growing in your body, makes this truly a nine-month journey, a time many women remember as special, one that never loses its place in their lives.

And "just being pregnant" is full of details. Specifics about how you feel on a daily basis: nauseated and tired, or bursting with energy; vulnerable and weepy, or simply ebullient; dumpy and fat, or proud of your newly voluptuous body. You wonder if you're eating the right foods, if you're taking in enough of them, if you're gaining too much weight. There are precautions to learn about, signs to be on the alert for, and tests to take to check for problems.

Then there's the day you really *know* yourself to be a *pregnant woman*. There's seeing or hearing your baby's heartbeat at your prenatal visits, and there's feeling him or her move inside your body for the first time. The comfortable hands-on-the-belly position when sitting becomes an instinctive, intimate gesture of protectiveness and of connection between mother and baby in utero.

But back to the details. In Part Two we'll take a straightforward look at how your baby grows and how your pregnancy progresses month by month. The information is organized like this: Each month starts with a list of the highlights of your baby's development. Second, the monthly progress of some of the best-known, most conspicuous features is charted; and third, any other particularly notable ones for that period of weeks are also touched upon. Last is a "topic of the month" segment that focuses on a specific common question or concern. (In Appendix A, titled, "Should I Worry?" you'll find information on potential danger signals during pregnancy.)

Here is a preview of the topics we'll look at: your due date, nausea, routine prenatal care, weight gain, exercise, full term-postterm-preterm, breastfeeding or bottle feeding, packing for the hospital and preparing for a newborn, and signs of labor and pain medication.

The First Trimester

THE FIRST MONTH: CONCEPTION—4.5 WEEKS

Baby

- Growth begins almost as soon as you conceive when the fertilized egg divides into two cells less than thirty minutes later.[1]

- Cell division continues while your fertilized egg (called a *zygote*)[2] makes its way through your fallopian tube and into your uterus to implant.

- Implantation takes place in the wall of your uterus five to seven days after conception.[3]

- With implantation, conception is now complete.[4]

- With implantation, the placenta begins to develop and your developing baby is now called an *embryo*.[5]

- The amniotic sac begins to form.[6]

- Heart, lungs, and central nervous system (the baby's brain and spinal cord) begin to develop.[7]

- Before you may even know you are pregnant, the baby's tiny heart is actually beating and circulating blood.[8]

- Rudimentary organs are in place.[9]

- Arm and leg buds are discernible.[10]

- Eyes and ears are starting to develop.[11]

- By the end of month one, the embryo weighs less than ⅓ ounce and measures a tiny ¼ to ½ inch.[12]

Mother

- Breast tenderness and a slight increase in breast size are often the first signs of pregnancy. Some women have the same feeling of fullness and tenderness they normally do before a period comes; for others there are no really noticeable changes outside of a missed period until the fifth or sixth week or even later in pregnancy.

- Nausea and fatigue may be a clue even this early that you have conceived.

• Frequent urination can be another clue in the first month of pregnancy, although those women who urinate more with a pending period won't be certain this symptom is actually another piece of evidence until later.

• Your appetite might change in the first month even without the presence of any nausea, making you more selective about your food choices. Changes, if any, may be incremental, or you may find yourself craving certain foods or find former favorites surprisingly unappealing. Some women experience a metallic type of taste in their mouth.[13]

Notables

• No period, sometimes a very light flow or spotting.

• Implantation cramp. Some women experience a mild ache or twinges when the embryo imbeds in the uterine wall. Sometimes implantation causes spotting.

• A feeling that something is subtly different.

• Nothing noticeably different at all other than a missed or light period.

• A positive pregnancy test. Fourteen days after conception is probably the "earliest-best" point to get an accurate result.[14] Pregnancy is confirmed when the amount of the hormone HCG reaches a certain level. The level of this hormone varies from woman to woman; some have a greater amount of HCG present earlier in their pregnancies than do others. The level of HCG in your blood might be enough for a positive pregnancy test as soon as seven days after conception, and in your urine at ten days after you've conceived. Pregnancy is typically confirmed with a urine test at ten to fourteen days after conception.[15]

Your Due Date

Pregnancy actually lasts about thirty-eight weeks, or 266 days, counting from the day you conceive through birth.[16] Since the day of conception is often not known, however, most obstetricians count the first day of your last period as the first day of pregnancy. Based on the average cycle length of twenty-eight days, adding on those fourteen days between ovulation and menstruation, makes a total of forty, weeks or 280 days. This is just over nine months of pregnancy[17] with a month being approximately 4.3 weeks long.

Dating a pregnancy two weeks older than it is in fact may strike you as a little peculiar. Plus, if you have been practicing fertility awareness or are otherwise certain of the day you ovulate, you'll probably be able to come close to pinpointing the moment you conceive. However, the standard method of determining the age of your pregnancy is very important to bear in mind.

The routine care you receive prenatally, including both pregnancy tests and monitoring of your progress (your weight gain, the baby's heartbeat and movement, all apparent and happening within the range of normal), as well as when prenatal diagnostic tests are scheduled, are most often guided by this standard dating process.

To calculate the day your baby is due, add seven to the date of the first day of your last menstrual period. Count back three months from that number and then count forward one full year.[18] So if your last period began on November 16, add 7, to make 23. Count back 3 months, to August 23, and add one year.

Only about 5 percent of babies are born the precise day they are due, which is also called the *estimated date of delivery*, or *EDD*, or *estimated date of confinement* or *EDC*. Most babies are born within a range that spans two weeks on either side.[19]

THE SECOND MONTH: 4.5 - 9 WEEKS

Baby

- The baby's spinal cord and brain are now well formed.[20]

- Close to the end of this month, the heart will be robustly beating and pumping blood.[21] At six weeks it may be visible in an ultrasound exam.

- The beginnings of hands and feet appear on leg and arm buds.[22]

- Organs are forming.[23]

- By the end of the month, the embryo will have a human-looking face, with the formation of eyes, ears, nose, cheeks, lips, and tongue.[24] The beginnings of a mouth and jaw are evident.[25]

- By the end of month two, the embryo will weigh about ⅓ ounce and be around 1 to 2 inches in length.[26]

Mother

- Breast changes are probably obvious this month. The breasts can be very sensitive to the touch; a very slight bump or a little bit of pressure, or even gently drying off with a towel can be painful. Nipples and areola may darken, and nipples along with the tiny bumps surrounding them may become more prominent. (These are glands that produce a substance that protects your breast during breastfeeding).[27] The network of veins under the skin may become more visible. Breasts are fuller, heavier. You may experience a tingling sensation.

- Nausea usually begins or may increase if already present, although not all women will experience it.

- Fatigue may be noticeable now, or continue from the time it began last month. You may feel a constant, bone-deep exhaustion or simply have less interest and energy to get up and go.

- You are probably urinating more frequently and it is clearly not associated with your period being due at this point.

- Appetite changes may be more obvious, craving certain foods, repelled by others.

Notables

- Before your pregnancy shows, your waist first begins to thicken. If not before, this month you'll probably notice that your clothes are tighter than they were around the middle.[28]

- Some women experience uterine or deep abdominal twinges beginning early and lasting throughout gestation. Although not necessarily danger signals, (when they might be is discussed in Appendix A) both twinging and contractions should be brought to your physician's attention and should be self-monitored.

Uterine twinges can originate from the constant activity in and around the uterus, which includes the baby's growth, the enlargement of the uterus, and the anatomical accommodations thus required. Some women have a sensitive, irritable uterus that seems to register more of the incredible physical activity that is involved in a growing pregnancy.

Nausea

Morning sickness in pregnancy ranges from mild to severe and can occur at any time of day or night, not just in the morning. Some women hardly suffer any obvious nausea at all; rather than nausea, their morning sickness takes the form of minor food or odor aversions. Others are moderately queasy for several hours per day, with perhaps a daily window of time during which they feel nearly normal. About 50 percent of women vomit during pregnancy,[29] a few—about 1 in 72—so often they need to be hospitalized.[30] *Hyperemesis gravidarum* is a pregnancy condition involving nearly total intolerance of any food or drink and persistent vomiting that can lead to dehydration and severe weight loss. A weight loss in the neighborhood of 5 percent or more of your pre-pregnancy weight is typically the point of concern.[31]

Few women are totally unaffected by morning sickness in the first trimester,[32] almost all falling somewhere within this fairly broad range as described above. Both common and universal, it is part of the pregnancies of women living all over the world,[33] regardless of how untouched the culture or how tranquil or natural the physical environment. Many women feel better around the time they are starting into their fourth month,[34] although about 25 percent are still feeling sick by twenty weeks, with some experiencing morning sickness throughout all forty weeks.[35]

Nausea in early pregnancy is commonly thought to be a good sign that a pregnancy is viable and going strong. Yet the opposite is also true, and the lack of nausea does not necessarily signal trouble. The cause of morning sickness is not known, but many theories about it boil down to the varied effects on the body of the flood of hormones produced beginning with conception.

These hormone-induced changes are theorized to include a heightened sense of smell,[36] explaining the reflexive nausea many women experience in the vicinity of previously benign, everyday odors. Now workplace smells, public restrooms, and even home bathrooms, your husband's breath or body odor, the smell of certain foods, and even perfumes can trigger waves of feeling sick and/or vomiting.

Although you probably already knew that feeling sick is normal in pregnancy, you may worry that the nausea or vomiting, or your inability to eat the recommended foods and portions, are creating a poor start for your baby. And of course you want some help in feeling better.

First, neither nausea, vomiting (unless you become dehydrated, for instance, and do not receive any treatment)[37], a short-lived minimal diet, or a decidedly unbalanced diet temporarily adapted while a pregnant woman's appetite is so delicate, appear to create problems for a developing baby.[38] In fact, evolutionary biologist Margie Profet approaches "pregnancy sickness" as an innate protective mechanism functioning to prevent a woman from eating foods with toxin levels that could harm the vulnerable fetus during the first few months of pregnancy.[39]

The best course in terms of managing your morning sickness may well be the most reasonable one, as follows: Do the very best you can in maintaining a pregnancy diet that includes all the important nutrients—folate, calcium, iron, and so on. Continue, if possible, taking your prenatal vitamins or consult your doctor about a more palatable, temporary option if they make you sick. And trust your body.

This last means that during the weeks you are experiencing nausea or vomiting, eating what you think will make you feel better, and doing so at the time you want that food, may be more effective than the usual crackers/ginger ale/hard candy recommendations.

In her book *No More Morning Sickness,* author Miriam Erick mentions lemonade, Tootsie Rolls, and potato chips among the foods her hospitalized patients asked for. Women who were given *what* they wanted to eat, *when* they wanted it, had the best results in minimizing their nausea and vomiting.[40]

Some pregnant women crave items that are nonfoods, such as dirt, clay, and chalk. This is called *pica.* It is important that you *not* follow any urges to eat such items, but do speak with your doctor about these cravings so that they can be evaluated.

As always, consult your physician about any concerns or questions you have about your nausea, vomiting, food intake, or food choices.

THE THIRD MONTH: 9 - 13.5 WEEKS

Baby

- This month, legs develop knees,[41] and arms, hands, fingers, feet, and toes will fully form.[42]

- Fingernails, toenails, and teeth are beginning to develop.[43]

- Liver, kidneys, gallbladder, pancreas and digestive and thyroid glands now actually begin to function.[44]

- The baby can swallow and suck by the end of the month.[45]

- Sperm are present in the testes if a boy, eggs in a girl.[46]

- Hair may grow on the baby's head.[47]

- The baby is very active, stretching, waving arms and legs, but the movements are not yet strong enough to be felt.[48]

- The baby's heartbeat can be heard this month with an instrument called a *Doppler*, usually around twelve weeks of pregnancy.[49]

- Genitals may be evident on ultrasound.[50]

- Around ten weeks of pregnancy (eight weeks after conception), the developing baby is no longer an embryo, but is now (and until birth) officially called a *fetus*.[51]

- By the end of month three, the developing baby will weigh about 1 ounce and be around 4 inches long.[52]

Mother

- Breasts may still feel tender and be increasing in size, although for some women the incredible breast growth and the sensitivity that comes with it slows during this month as they come to the end of their first trimester. A bra that fits you at this point will probably work for the rest of your pregnancy as long as it can be adjusted to allow for the increase in back size of the later months.[53] Also *colostrum* production may begin.[54] (See next month for more on this "pre-milk.")

- Nausea may be gone by the end of this month for many women.[55] Fatigue may also begin to abate. Urination varies from woman to woman, but may begin to be less frequent.

- Cravings and food aversions may continue, but during this month some women find their appetite is returning and they are beginning to tolerate a wider range of foods.

Notables

- The later part of this month, you may begin to "show," with the appearance of a gentle swelling in the area between your pubic bone and navel.[56]

- Most miscarriages occur within the first trimester. Although not a guarantee of a safe passage all the way through pregnancy, reaching your tenth week with the baby's heartbeat and movement seen via an ultrasound examination is a positive sign.[57]

- This is the month to have chorionic villus sampling (ten to twelve weeks) for those women choosing this procedure for prenatal diagnosis.

- Early amniocentesis may be scheduled during this month, usually not before your twelfth week.

Routine Prenatal Care

Your doctor will ask you to take several routine tests during the course of your prenatal care. Some are done only once, while others are done at every regular appointment. The information below will give you an idea of the kind of tests typically involved in monitoring your pregnancy.

Blood tests checking for:

Blood type—First visit.[58]

Rh factor—First visit.[59] When the mother has Rh negative blood, and the father is positive for Rh, the fetus may inherit the positive Rh factor. A blood incompatibility can develop, causing the mother's body to make antibodies that attack her developing baby's blood. Either the fetus or newborn can become seriously ill or die as a result. This allergic-like reaction usually doesn't pose a danger during a first pregnancy because the antibodies in the mother's blood are slow to develop; it does, however, endanger subsequent pregnancies. Special measures may be taken now to safeguard your future pregnancies, as well as to ensure the fetus is not harmed in your current one.[60]

Anemia—First visit and at twenty-eight weeks.[61] When there are too few red blood cells in the blood, the volume of oxygen carried in it is decreased. Anemia is most commonly the result of an iron deficiency; fatigue, dizziness, pale skin, and insomnia are among the symptoms. During gestation, blood volume increases tremendously to support the growing fetus, making pregnant women more likely to become anemic. Anemia occurs most frequently later in pregnancy.[62]

Syphilis and Hepatitis B, sometimes chlamydia and gonorrhea—First visit.[63] All these sexually transmitted diseases can seriously affect the babies of infected mothers. Syphilis can cause a miscarriage or stillbirth if it passes from the mother's blood into the fetus. A baby born with syphilis may have hearing defects or be blind or deformed, among a multitude of other problems.[64]

Hepatitis B is picked up by the majority of the babies (80 percent) born to infected mothers. Usually infected during birth, most of these infants will become lifelong carriers of this virus. Carriers may go on to develop serious conditions such as cirrhosis or hardening of the liver, and can pass the virus to others.[65]

The two most common of all the sexually transmitted diseases, chlamydia and gonorrhea, are both caused by bacteria. Babies become exposed during delivery; chlamydia can cause eye infections and pneumonia in a newborn, and gonorrhea can cause eye infections that could lead to blindness if untreated. Almost all newborns receive eye drops to prevent infection by the gonococcal bacteria.[66]

Rubella and mumps immunity—First/early visit.[67] These tests show whether you have the antibodies that will protect you from becoming infected with the rubella or mumps virus.

A baby exposed to rubella (German measles) in utero may be born deaf, with cataracts (an eye condition that can progress to blindness), heart disease, or mental retardation. The fetus is most vulnerable to developing birth defects when the mother contracts the rubella virus within the first three months.[68] The earlier she is infected in the course of pregnancy, the greater the chance the baby will be born with problems.[69]

Mumps double the risk for a miscarriage if an expectant mother is infected within her first twelve weeks, and it has also been linked to preterm labor.[70] Your immunity to mumps and rubella should be checked early in your prenatal care[71] if not included in the panel of tests done on the blood drawn at your initial visit.

Toxoplasmosis—First visit.[72] You will be tested for the presence of antibodies that give you immunity to toxoplasmosis, an infection caused by a parasite. Birth defects can result when a woman becomes infected for the first time while she is pregnant.[73] This disease can cause jaundice, fever, blindness, hydrocephaly (fluid on the brain), and mental retardation.[74] While the growing baby in utero is most susceptible to toxoplasmosis during the last trimester, she or he is more likely to develop severe problems when a woman becomes infected within the first twelve weeks of pregnancy.[75]

Gestational Diabetes—at twenty-four to twenty-eight weeks. Checking for high levels of glucose, which might signal the development of gestational diabetes.

Urine tests checking for:
Protein—Every visit. High levels may be a sign of pregnancy-induced hypertension (preeclampsia).[76] When a woman with this condition does not receive treatment, a lower birth weight

or spontaneous premature birth may result.[77] An early induced or surgical delivery may also be advised, depending on the danger posed to mother and baby by continuing the pregnancy.[78] Although most often preeclampsia can be treated successfully,[79] a condition not brought under control can become so severe as to endanger the mother's life—although fortunately, this happens only rarely.[80]

Glucose—Every visit. High levels may be a sign of gestational diabetes.[81] When this condition is not controlled, the babies of these mothers may be *macrosomic*, which means they grow to be overly large. With weights of approximately 10 pounds and even higher, these babies are more difficult to deliver.[82]

Other tests:
Pelvic exam—First visit. General examination of your reproductive organs, plus looking for changes in the cervix that occur with pregnancy as well as in the uterus and pelvis.[83] Usually not done again until close to the end of gestation to reduce the risk of introducing infection or otherwise harming your pregnancy.

Ultrasound—Throughout, depending on your physician's practice protocol as well as any individual risk factors. Vaginal sonograms may be done until the pregnancy advances far enough so that transabdominal ultrasound is needed for a full view of the baby.[84] A fetal heartbeat may be checked every visit beginning around twelve weeks, when it can be heard with the use of a Doppler (a hand-held ultrasound type of device that translates motion into sound). A detailed, complete sonogram may be done after eighteen weeks.[85]

Your weight gain, blood pressure, and uterine expansion will be checked regularly. Other tests may be done if called for, for example, because of family history or any problems cropping up at any point during pregnancy.

Your appointment schedule may look something like this:[86]

Once every four weeks through twenty-seven weeks.

Once every two weeks from twenty-eight through thirty-five weeks.

Once a week at thirty-six weeks until birth.

The Second Trimester

THE FOURTH MONTH: 13.5–18 WEEKS

Baby

- All the organs, the body systems, and body parts are formed by fourteen weeks. The greater period of vulnerability to severe harm to these body structures from teratogens or poor diet will then have passed.[87]

- Hands can now grasp.[88]

- Feet can move and toes can wiggle.[89]

- The skin is transparent.[90]

- The baby has eyebrows and eyelashes.[91]

- The baby may suck on his or her thumb.[92]

- The baby will weigh about 8 ounces and be around 6 to 7 inches in length by eighteen weeks.[93]

Mother

- Breasts become less firm, tenderness lessens. The baby's first, ultra-nutritious and beneficial food, called *colostrum*, begins to be made in the breast as early as twelve to fourteen weeks.[94] Some women actually produce colostrum as early as month five,[95] others not until after delivery, when this sticky, yellowish fluid feeds the baby before your milk comes in.[96]

- Nausea decreases and ends for many women by the time their fourteenth week begins.[97]

- Fatigue often lessens. Some women feel vital and healthy during their middle trimester.

- Urination varies. It may be less than in the first trimester, but still more than prepregnancy.

- Appetite may bloom. Especially after months of aversions and nausea, food may be experienced as an enormous pleasure.

Notables

- Your heart will pump 30 percent to 50 percent more blood while you are pregnant, an increase that peaks during this month and remains high until the thirtieth week.[98] The total volume of blood circulating in your body also increases.[99] The upgraded cardiovascular activity translates into a facial flush, a radiant, pregnancy "glow" that many women experience in these middle weeks.

- Either early amniocentesis (before fifteen weeks) or standard amniocentesis (fifteen to eighteen weeks) can be done this month.

- The multiple marker screening test is accurate between fifteen and twenty weeks, although targeting weeks sixteen to seventeen falling in your fourth month, is suggested. (See section on MMS in Chapter Three.)

- The alpha fetoprotein test is also done at fifteen to twenty weeks, with sixteen to seventeen weeks recommended. (See the section on AFP in Chapter Three.)

Weight Gain

The amount of weight your doctor recommends you gain will depend in part on your prepregnancy weight.[100] Gaining 25 to 35 pounds is a typical range if you are beginning pregnancy at a normal weight. Somewhat more, 28 to 40 pounds, may be advised if you are underweight, with an even larger gain for a woman carrying twins, 35 to 45 pounds. The range drops down to 15 to 25 pounds if you are overweight, and 15 pounds is recommended for obese women.

Dieting and pregnancy don't mix—something vital to your baby's development and your health (such as folic acid or calcium) can easily be shortchanged. So, at the lower ends of weight gain, it is especially important to maintain an optimal pregnancy diet even with some limits on calorie intake. All pregnant women, however, do want to make "nutrient dense" food choices as much as possible. These are foods that provide necessary nutrients and may give you the advantage of satisfying multiple nutrition requirements. For instance, milk provides protein and calcium along with several vitamins and minerals, most of which are valuable during pregnancy.[101] The right weight gain and food plan for you should be discussed at your first prenatal visit.

Providing the brand-new embryo/fetus with vitamins and minerals important to early development is really the emphasis of this initial period when its tiny organs are just forming.[102] Nutrient needs, such as iron, protein, and calcium, and, early on, especially folate, increase much more than do calorie needs.[103] In fact, you need only about 100 additional calories per day in the first three months, and even in your second and third trimester, only about a total of 300 more calories per day are required.[104]

The increase in calories translates into a per month rate of weight gain around 2 to 4 pounds in your first trimester, then ¾ to 1 pound per week until birth.[105]

Your total pregnancy weight gain is a function of more than your baby's size and putting on fat.[106] For example, your breasts, uterus, and amniotic fluid may each weigh about 2 pounds, the placenta about 1.5 pounds, and the weight of both the augmented fluid and blood volume in your body may now be 4 pounds each. Your nutrient stores may be around 7 pounds, and the baby, on average, 7.5 pounds. Of this combined 30 pounds, you will immediately lose about 11 with the birth of your baby, which includes his or her weight, along with that of the placenta and amniotic fluid.[107]

Although gaining enormous amounts of weight can cause problems—for instance by increasing the possibility of developing gestational diabetes—gaining insufficient weight may lead to an undernourished, low-birthweight baby. Weighing 5.5 pounds or under, these babies often have complications that are life-threatening.[108] Eating well and gaining adequate weight is one way to very much lessen your chances of having a low birthweight baby.

For the woman who misses her thinner, smaller, prepregnant body terribly, it can take some time to adjust to an ever-expanding and transforming shape. Yet the bodily rounding and softening that comes with your weight gain is unalterable, as the added fat tissue is actually functional in pregnancy.

Pregnancy hormones change the way your body metabolizes food, and even very lean women will accumulate fat during pregnancy.[109] Fat stores (with their reserves of calories and nutrients) are actually more easily created, ready to be called upon if food intake drops dangerously low and in preparation for breast-feeding. Your body will draw from these stores in the process of producing milk—a process that requires even more calories than pregnancy![110]

Most of us do come to accept our changed body image at some point during the nine months. Sooner or later we grow comfortable, and some, even pleased by the fullness of their shape as a pregnant woman.

THE FIFTH MONTH: 18–22.5 WEEKS

Baby

- The baby's skin will be covered this month by *lanugo*, a fine downy hair that is mostly shed before the last month of pregnancy.[111] Sometimes patches of lanugo are still present at birth, but they fall off soon after.

- A creamy, whitish substance called *vernix* protects the baby's skin in utero and may still coat the baby at birth.[112]

- Eyelids may be able to open and close.[113]

- Genitals are now evident; you can see what sex your baby is with ultrasound.[114]

- He or she now looks much like a miniature baby[115] with wrinkly, translucent skin.[116]

- This month the baby weighs in at about 1 pound and is around 9 inches long.[117]

Mother

- Your breasts are probably no longer excruciatingly tender or painful, but may be more sensitive to accidental bumps than they were prepregnancy. Colostrum may begin to leak from your breasts this month.[118]

- Nausea will be gone for most women.[119]

- Urination may be less than in the first trimester, but more than prepregnancy.[120]

- Appetite is hardy, food may be a surprising focus during your day.

Notables

- Fetal movement or "quickening" may be felt as early as fourteen weeks,[121] but most women first sense movement between sixteen and twenty weeks.[122] The earliest movements are subtle. They may feel like the lightest flicker of a touch deep inside your body, often described as butterflies in your stomach, or as a tickling or a fluttering sensation. Your movement is soothing to the baby; he or she may be lulled to sleep when you're active and be much busier when you're resting.

- Your pregnancy will become obvious by around twenty weeks, when your belly swells around the navel area.[123]

- Round ligament pain occurs most often between eighteen and twenty-four weeks.[124] This sharp or achy feeling in your lower abdomen or groin happens when the ligaments that support your uterus begin to stretch. If the pain becomes more severe, or comes and goes regularly (every ten minutes, for example), you should call your doctor immediately.

Exercise During Pregnancy

Regular activity may not only reduce some of the physical discomforts of pregnancy,[125] but contributes to a feeling of well-being and will help you maintain a sense of connection with your body—no small feat when your physical transformation is so dramatic.

However, the hormones of pregnancy create changes that call for extra care during exercise. For instance, your ligaments soften, your joints become more movable, and pain and injuries are thus more likely.[126] And of course your balance changes as your baby grows, making you more susceptible to falls.

The overriding guideline is to *listen to your body*. Wait until after you have the baby to push yourself to your limits, or to maintain a rigorous exercise schedule even when you feel fatigued. Go with the signals your body gives you. Ease up on the intensity when your energy level begins to drop, pass on exercises that cause even a tiny bit of strain anywhere in your body, and stop when you're tired.

Here are some specific suggestions adapted from standards set by the American College of Obstetricians and Gynecologists (ACOG).[127] These general guidelines will help you exercise safely. Exercise has by and large been found to be safe during pregnancy, but be sure to speak with your physician about your standard exercise routine to individualize a plan that may include more or fewer limitations.

EXERCISE GUIDELINES

TYPE

• Avoid high impact aerobics and other jarring forms of exercise. Be judicious and cautious about participating in sports where you are vulnerable to falling or susceptible to injury, such as horseback riding, skiing, and soccer. Avoid water skiing and surfing completely because of the danger a hard, fast fall poses to both an expectant mother and her baby. Instead try walking, swimming (but not scuba diving), and low-impact aerobics. Runners and joggers should speak with their doctor about continuing in pregnancy if this is already part of their regular workout.

• Avoid exercises that create stress on your back or knees, such as deep knee bends, straight leg sit-ups, and double leg lifts.

• After your twentieth week do not do exercises lying on your back for more than a minute or two. Some experts are even more cautious, recommending no exercise flat on your back after the first trimester.[128] Your uterus, now larger and heavier, may rest on the large vein lying beneath it in this position. The amount of blood your heart can pump might be reduced, effectively decreasing the flow of blood to the uterus.

• Stretch easily rather than extending all the way to your limits to help prevent injury.

FREQUENCY

• Exercise regularly, three times per week or more. If you do not already have an exercise routine, you'll want to build up gradually and carefully during pregnancy. Speak with your doctor about developing a personalized exercise plan.

OVERHEATING

• Avoid overheating. Your body temperature should remain under 101 degrees. You can get an idea of how high yours rises by taking your temperature (an underarm temperature is recommended) after a typical workout; thereafter use that measurement as a guide to monitor and modify the intensity of your effort. Alternatively, exercise lightly in hot, humid weather. Drinking plenty of water (to minimize the risk of dehydration) will help you keep your temperature down. Be careful about using hot tubs and saunas after working out (or at any time during pregnancy), but especially during the first trimester.

DURATION AND INTENSITY

• Keep to a maximum of thirty minutes of intense exercise if you were active and fit before you conceived. Otherwise, limit it to fifteen to twenty minutes.

• Begin and end all vigorous workouts with at least five to ten minutes of warm-up exercises and stretches.

WATER

• Drink water before, during, and after exercise. Don't wait until you're thirsty; rather, keep yourself regularly hydrated.

EQUIPMENT

• Wear a supportive bra and well-fitting, cushioned shoes.

DANGER SIGNALS

Stop exercising if you:

• Feel pain of any sort, especially in your back, pubic area, or uterus (cramping).

- Begin bleeding from your vagina.

- Notice your heat beating abnormally—either rapidly or irregularly.

- Feel dizzy, faint, or short of breath.

- Have problems with walking.

Call your physician to report any of these symptoms. You'll also want additional advice about the safest course from this point onward about your level of exercise.

Your first prenatal visit is a good time to talk about exercise during pregnancy. There are certain conditions where you may be advised against either vigorous or perhaps even mild exercise, for instance if you are at risk for premature labor. Ask your physician about your individual risk.

THE SIXTH MONTH: 22.5–27 WEEKS

Baby

- The baby can now hear noises inside your body and some that are outside. Loud noises might startle him or her.[129]

- The hair on the baby's head may now be growing.[130]

- The baby may get the hiccups.[131]

- The baby may suck on her or his thumb.[132]

- Fingernails, toenails, and bones are hardening.[133]

- Skin is becoming opaque.[134]

- The baby's weight this month is about 1.5 pounds and length is usually between 11 and 14 inches.[135]

Mother

- You may notice that your breasts have grown slightly in size and that you are showing more than you were even a couple of weeks ago. Your nausea is probably long past, and you are still energetic, although you may suddenly "cross the line" unawares, become surprisingly tired, and need to rest. Compared to the burst of physical developments in the first trimester, the changes during these middle months are more gradual, progressing at something of an unhurried pace.

Notables

- Twenty-four weeks is generally considered the lowest limit of fetal viability.[136] Enough development has been completed at twenty-four weeks, that about 15 to 20 percent of babies born at this point will live when treated in a modern neonatal intensive care unit.[137] The down side is that few will emerge without damage related to preterm birth. These babies often end up with lifelong neurological problems, such as visual impairment or cerebral palsy.[138]

Full Term—Postterm—Preterm

A baby born between thirty-seven and forty-two weeks is a *full-term* baby—and most are, with 80 percent delivered within this rather wide span of time.[139] Only about 5 percent are delivered precisely on the date they are due—most women give birth at some point during the two weeks before or after this date.[140] Pregnancy lasts approximately forty weeks (280 days or about 9.3 calendar months), on average, from the first day of your last period, or about thirty-eight weeks (266 days or around 8.8 calendar months), from the day of conception.[141]

When pregnancy lasts beyond forty-two weeks it is called a *postterm* pregnancy. Although less than one in ten of these late-late babies have any gestation-length related problems, your doctor will probably begin to more closely evaluate and monitor your baby's health at forty-one to forty-two weeks.[142] About 10 percent of pregnancies are postterm and approximately 10 percent of births are *preterm*.[143] When labor and delivery occur before your thirty-seventh week, it is considered preterm.[144]

Most of the time the cause of a preterm delivery is not known[145] and many such deliveries occur among women whose pregnancies appeared to be utterly normal.[146] It is truly amazing that a tiny six-month-old fetus may actually have a chance to live, but those who do usually have access to aggressive medical intervention in a modern intensive care unit; even with the best of care, these children will often have long-term neurological difficulties that are associated with prematurity.[147]

Nevertheless, your twenty-fourth week is still the crossroads in terms of fetal viability, and the picture of course gets better from there: With only one additional week of gestation, a premie's survival rate leaps from 15 to 20 percent up to 50 to 60 percent at 25 weeks; then even higher, up to 85 percent, for weeks twenty-six to twenty-eight and over 90 percent at twenty-nine weeks.[148] The *pivotal* point in the course of your pregnancy is at thirty-two weeks.[149] Typically a child born at this time survives without any health problems caused by arriving early. Prior to thirty-two weeks, many babies have not yet produced a vital substance called *surfactant*. Without surfactant, he or she may need intensive medical care to support breathing—including oxygen and respirators. While a baby born at thirty-two-plus weeks will still need intensive care, the chance for survival is 95 percent or better, and the overwhelming majority live to be normal and healthy.

The Third Trimester

THE SEVENTH MONTH: 27–31.5 WEEKS

Baby
- The baby sucks his or her thumb often.[150]

- His or her lanugo starts shedding.[151]

- This month the baby will probably turn upside down in your uterus.[152]

- The baby is larger now and has much less room to move. The tighter fit makes his or her movements more visible to the eye and more palpable under your hand or that of another person gently resting on your belly.[153]

- His or her body is nearly fully developed.[154]

- A layer of fat is forming under the skin and the baby is beginning to plump up.[155]

- The baby weighs about 2.5 to 3 pounds this month and is between 14 and 17 inches long.[156]

Mother

- Fatigue may increase but probably won't be the constant, bone-deep type of weariness of your first trimester.

- Your appetite may become more "delicate." Your digestive system is not only functioning less efficiently, but your intestines are being crowded as your uterus expands.[157] You may find yourself becoming more discerning in your food choices and eating less at each sitting.

- The feeling of needing to urinate may increase as your growing uterus presses against your bladder.

Notables

- Many women now become aware of irregular uterine contractions. Called *Braxton-Hicks* contractions, they usually start sometime in your first trimester, then increase in intensity throughout gestation.[158] Braxton-Hicks usually become recognizable around your seventh or eighth month.[159] They may be hard to distinguish from actual labor pains when the end of pregnancy is approaching.[160] We'll soon look at when early contractions could signal premature labor.

- Your stomach, intestines, bladder, diaphragm, and other organs are displaced and squeezed together as your expanding uterus takes up more and more room.[161] Only in pregnancy would this distorted conformation of your internal organs be considered normal!

Breastfeeding Versus Bottle Feeding

There is no question that breastfeeding your baby can be a wonderful experience; utterly maternal, fulfilling, deeply bonding, tender, and intimate—the list is long for those women who have mostly positive feelings about nursing. Providing your own child with nourishment is for many women a part of childcare they cherish.

The medical facts about nursing are also positive. Breast milk contains antibodies and other factors that provide your new baby with immunological protection against a number of viral and bacterial infections,[162] discouraging colds and other illnesses. Colostrum, the liquid that is produced in your breasts before your milk comes in, is particularly high in protective antibodies.[163]

Breast milk also contains a perfectly balanced blend of ingredients, a mixture that changes in response to variations in your baby's nutritional needs.[164] In addition, nursing speeds up postpartum weight loss for some women[165] because of the calories the body expends in making milk.

The pluses of breastfeeding are indeed worthwhile and do deserve thoughtful consideration as you decide whether to nurse. Yet there are drawbacks to be aware of. For instance, while many women experience mild nipple soreness from time to time when nursing, for some the pain can be intense. Even if you properly position the baby on your breast, (called *latching on*) and take other measures to ease the problem, discomfort can still develop.

Women who work outside the home may need to take extra measures when it comes to breastfeeding. Some women use a breast pump to collect their milk, which a caregiver then feeds to the baby while they're gone. Others bring a pump with them and use it at work, keeping the milk in an insulated container along with an ice pack, as breast milk should not be stored at room temperature. Many women combine breast and bottle feeding, nursing before and after work and using formula for the baby's meals during the day. While there are a number of options that will work, individual circumstances can make the extra measures required impractical for some working mothers.

Fortunately, while breastfeeding will give your baby's health an early boost, your child's well-being does not hang on being breastfed. Further, there is so much involved in the totality of mothering that the gratification you receive in caring for your baby and the depth of the bond between you and your child by no means hinges on whether you nurse.

In fact, bottle feeding has its own kind of emotional fullness. A bottle feeding mother makes the formula, she might test the temperature on her inner forearm, and then hold the bottle with care in her child's mouth while he or she drinks. The image of a mother holding her baby close to her body during meals, stroking, talking softly, or absorbed in simply watching, is time-honored. The whole bottle preparation and feeding process is a motherly ritual, one that can be rich, loving, and giving.

Whichever choice *feels best* and *fits best* for you is the right one. Your doctor, nurse practitioner, or midwife can give you further information about the medical and practical, pluses and minuses of both nursing and bottle feeding. One last note, however. If you are planning on breastfeeding, you want to be sure your nipples are not inverted or flat, making it hard for the baby to latch onto your breast. Your nipples can be drawn out with the use of breast shells. Check with your prenatal care provider early in pregnancy if you have any concerns that yours don't protrude enough or at all.

THE EIGHTH MONTH: 31.5 WEEKS–36 WEEKS

Baby

- The baby now needs to accumulate just another layer of fat for warmth and a little more lung development to be ready for breathing independently when born.[166]

- His or her skin is more pink in color.[167]

- This month, the baby weighs about 3.5 to 6 pounds and is between 16 and 18 inches in length.[168]

Mother

- Colostrum may leak from your breasts beginning this month if not before.[169] (Some women don't notice colostrum until after the baby is born.)

- You may feel tired and heavy from head to toe.

- Your appetite will probably continue to be more delicate than during your middle trimester; an increase in the feeling of needing to urinate often will probably continue as well.

Notables

- If your baby is born prematurely at thirty-two weeks or later, your chances of leaving the hospital with a normal, healthy baby in your arms are nevertheless, excellent.[170]

Packing for the Hospital/Preparing for a Newborn at Home

Packing for your stay at the hospital can be a fairly simple task. "Less is best" is the guideline many women are happiest with, especially when packing for the hospital happens all in a rush when the contractions first start or their water breaks. (While your first days at home with a new baby will indeed be much smoother if you have everything you need, more than a few of us never have a suitcase packed for the hospital and ready to be thrown in the car when it's finally time to go!) Below are the bare necessities, which should be more than enough:

For yourself:

- Change of clothes to come home in, comfortable for only a somewhat smaller body (you'll be about 11 pounds lighter).

- Nursing bra, or if not nursing, a bra with a roomy fit in the cups and back (to accommodate breasts engorged with milk).

- Hairbrush.

- Toothbrush.

- Toothpaste.

For the newborn:

- One onesie (also called a body suit), if weather is hot, or one lightweight sleeper, if cooler, or one blanket sleeper, if cold.

- Receiving blanket.

- Warm blanket in cold weather.

- Knit cap in cold weather.

- Car seat.

- Infant head support for car seat.

At home, ready for the new baby:
- Three onesies or sleepers.

- Diapers.

- Baby wipes.

- Diaper pail.

- Changing table.

- Changing pad.

- Crib.

- Crib mattress.

- Waterproof crib pad.

- Crib sheet.

- Wedge or tightly rolled towel to prop the baby on his or her side or back.

- Baby blanket.

- Bottles, unless nursing exclusively.

- Formula, unless nursing exclusively.

- Baby bath.

- Alcohol (umbilical cord care).

- Sterile 100 percent cotton balls (umbilical cord care).

THE NINTH MONTH: 36–40 WEEKS

Baby

- The baby's body is fuller and more rounded. He or she is still gaining weight, as much as an ounce per day.[171]

- His or her lungs are now mature.[172]

- Traces of lanugo may remain on the forehead, in front of the ears, and on the back, but most will have shed.[173]

- The vernix coating his or her skin begins to disappear[174] although the baby will probably still be coated at birth.[175]

- The larger rolling movements will be fewer now as the uterus is filled by the nine-month-old fetus. He or she may now be *engaged* in the pelvis. (See below in "Notables.") You will still feel the arms and legs moving around.[176]

- The baby weighs between 5.5 and 10 pounds this month and is 16.5 to 22 inches long.[177]

Mother

- At times during these last weeks, you may experience an unexpected increase in your energy level. You may find yourself possessed with making specific preparations for the baby, housecleaning, and finishing up work-related or other projects. However, not all women find themselves "preparing the nest" in this sort of purposeful way. In fact, many women are utterly uncomfortable and simply weary through most days of their ninth month of pregnancy.

- The feeling of needing to urinate will increase from the pressure on your bladder after the baby has dropped.

- Your appetite may vary from hungry all the time to a marked disinterest in eating.

Notables

- Now only weeks from giving birth, in response to some mysterious signal your body will make the transition from gestation toward labor. A woman pregnant for the first time may notice the baby's position has changed sometime between thirty-six and thirty-eight weeks.[178] During this time, the baby's head may drop into the pelvis, called *lightening*,[179] and become *engaged* or fixed against the cervix.[180] A second or later baby may not engage until labor begins.[181]

  Once the baby's head is engaged, your cervix will begin to *efface*, becoming shorter and thinning out from the action of your uterine contractions, and your cervix will start to *dilate* or widen, as the contractions cause the baby's head to push against it.[182] These steps occur either slowly and gradually over the entire ninth month or may begin even earlier. Sometimes they happen all at once in just hours as an immediate prelude to labor.[183]

- Another sign that might clue you to the possibility of labor approaching is the release of your *mucus plug*. A plug of mucus in the cervical canal has until now served as a protective barrier for the uterus during pregnancy. Also called *show*, you may or may not notice this small glop of either clear, pink, or reddish mucus (*bloody show*) loosened as your cervix dilates.[184]

Signs of Labor and Pain Medication

SIGNS OF LABOR

Some women show all the signs of labor approaching during their last month of pregnancy, while others may not experience any of them until their contractions begin, signaling the start of labor. Most women, however, notice one or more signs as they pass through their last weeks of pregnancy. Here is a summary of signals that labor is nearing;

- Braxton-Hicks contractions are stronger and more frequent.

- Lightening—the baby drops to a lower position in the pelvis.

- Engagement—the baby's head fixes deep in the pelvis against your cervix.

- Cervical effacement—your cervix shortens and thins.

- Cervical dilation—your cervix widens.

- Mucus plug is released as cervix dilates.

When you are in or very close to the onset of labor, in addition to any of those above, you may experience:[185]

- Rupture of membranes, more commonly spoken of as *your water breaks*.

- Contractions become regular, persistent, and progressive, meaning they increase in frequency, duration, and intensity (how often, how long, how bad).

False labor can be difficult to distinguish from real labor without an exam for telltale, progressive cervical changes. To help you discern which you are in, take note of your contractions as follows:[186]

- Are they regular or irregular? The Braxton-Hicks contractions of false labor are usually irregular.

- Are they persistent or sporadic? False labor contractions come and go rather than persisting and progressing. They may also fizzle if you change the position your body is in, if you take a walk after you've been resting, or, vice versa, if you rest after you've been on your feet.

- Are they progressive or nonprogressive? Typically only true labor contractions steadily, or sometimes abruptly, increase in frequency, duration, and intensity.

Generally speaking, you will be advised to go to the hospital sometime after true labor begins rather than at the very beginning. With a first baby, a typical recommendation is to wait until contractions come regularly every three to five minutes or less from the beginning of one to the start of the next, for a period of two hours; with a second or later child, every five to seven minutes or less for one hour.[187] Be sure to discuss with your doctor when you should go to the hospital.

You will usually also be advised to go to the hospital or at least call if these signs are present:[188]

- Vaginal bleeding.

- Ruptured membranes.

- Contractions that are severe and unrelenting, rather than the usual pattern of tightening, then release.

PAIN MEDICATION

Many women are curious about techniques that support a medication-free birth, even if they have no intention of going through labor without receiving drugs for pain relief. If this is so for you, or, conversely, if you plan to have your baby without medication, ask your physician or midwife where you can take a *childbirth preparation course.*

Typically, childbirth preparation classes provide a wealth of information about the birth process, often including details about pain medication options in addition to classroom time for practicing breathing and relaxation techniques. Sometimes you won't be able to receive medication during labor until some time after you request it—for instance, if you're not far enough along in labor. Individual physicians and hospitals vary in their criterion; some base the timing on how many centimeters dilated you are. Or the anesthesiologist may have other women waiting for medication ahead of you or be called in for an emergency cesarean that would take precedence over non-emergency needs for pain medication.

If they do have to wait for medication many women find the breathing and relaxation techniques helpful. Of the natural childbirth methods available, Lamaze, Bradley, and Dick-Read are the most popular. While education about the birth process itself is woven throughout all these methods, each has a different emphasis in approaching childbearing.

The best known is Lamaze. This method teaches a woman to respond to pain reflexively with specific breathing techniques to help her maintain control and provide a means of distraction during contractions.[189]

The Bradley method, in contrast, encourages a woman to keep her focus *inward* and *on her body*. Deep abdominal breathing techniques help a woman relax and go with the birth process. This approach also stresses the father's involvement throughout both pregnancy and birth.[190]

The oldest of the three is the Dick-Read method. Dr. Dick-Read introduced into the hospital delivery room the notion that education about the process of birth could be useful to laboring women. His philosophy that *ignorance-fear-tension-pain* are progressively linked during labor is the basis for childbirth preparation classes where women learn about the birth process, as well as how to deeply relax their bodies.[191]

Some women use natural childbirth techniques in conjunction with drugs, while others are able to cope well without first practicing any techniques. And for that matter, they may find ways of their own that take them through the entire course of labor without medication for pain relief.

Below you'll find brief descriptions of three types of drugs often used to ease pain during labor.

Demerol is an *analgesic,* a class of drugs that act systemically. Demerol will provide pain relief without causing you to lose consciousness. The degree of alleviation varies, usually lessening pain but not always banishing it entirely.[192]

Side effects also vary from woman to woman, and may involve feeling drowsy, dizzy, and nauseated. A newborn may emerge with usually short-term effects, including drowsiness and possibly weak respiration.[193]

An *epidural block* is a *regional anesthetic* administered in your low back, between the vertebra of your spinal cord. It effects the area extending from about your waist down. Continual pain medication can be received with an epidural as a small flexible tube called a *catheter* remains in place after the needle is withdrawn. Pain relief can range from more comfortable to the point of numbness.[194]

Some women have rejected epidurals because the numbness in their legs confined them to bed. However, a *walking epidural* is now in use in many hospitals, allowing a laboring woman to be mobile—believed to encourage the birth along—at the same time she experiences a significant reduction in pain. Check on the availability at the place you are planning on having your baby if you like the idea of an epidural.

Side effects for the mother may include difficulty in bearing down or pushing due to numbness and thus slowing down labor, as well as low blood pressure. The baby's heart rate may drop if the mother's blood pressure lowers.[195]

A *spinal block* is very similar to an epidural, including many of the side effects. One important difference is that pain medication is given only once with a spinal, rather than continuously as is possible with an epidural.[196] Another is that headaches are much more common.[197]

Your basic guidelines in choosing the pain medication you want during labor are (1) availability, and (2) getting the most relief with the mildest side effects for you and your baby.

Epilogue

The best time to have a baby is when you are emotionally, psychologically, and financially ready. Yet do keep in mind that sooner rather than later is the best advised course *fertility-wise* when it comes to getting pregnant, even if it takes just a little nudging to be right there.

It *is* important to factor in the time limits that exist on your fertility. You don't want to make plans for having a baby down the road, based on the *assumption* that you will still be able to conceive then. Of course, you can't know now if that will in fact be so.

In your mid-thirties, however, you have the good fortune of thinking about or trying to have a baby relatively young. Most often, being relaxed but focused is the right *initial* approach, with the physician-recommended six-month limit providing a kind of built-in back-up plan, just in case you don't conceive sooner. Even so, one blessing of still being in your thirties is a larger measure of time during which you'll be able to try.

As you get closer to and into your forties, the nearness of limits on your fertility creates the need for a more *purposeful* approach in trying to get pregnant. Forty-plus women take longer to conceive on average and miscarry more often as a group; sometimes pregnancy during these years can be something of a long-term project. The passing of months can really count, and it's wisest not to waste time.

While the picture would indeed be incomplete if a reader missed or minimized the notes of caution about fertility at midlife that are woven throughout this book, one of the main messages is that, nevertheless, yes, you *are* likely to get pregnant and have a baby in your mid- to late thirties and early forties.

May you conceive quickly and have an uneventful pregnancy. If you don't have a smooth course, don't give up until you know it's impossible, or are sure it's simply time for you to let it go, because having a baby is worth the effort. Best wishes to you for a wonderful midlife pregnancy.

Appendix A
Should I Worry?
Potential Danger Signs
During Pregnancy

BLEEDING-CONTRACTIONS-LACK OF FETAL MOVEMENT-HEADACHES

Some women worry only a little if at all about the safety of their pregnancies, and some do much more than their share, even when there are no signs to indicate theirs is anything but secure and robust. Wherever you might fall on the scale, it is important to be aware of those signs that might indicate a problem. The discussion that follows summarizes what to watch for.

BLEEDING

Vaginal bleeding during pregnancy is not necessarily a sign that your pregnancy is in jeopardy. However, the source of any bleeding needs to be assessed as quickly as possible in case a problem has developed or one is brewing that requires medical attention. Call your doctor if you notice any blood when you use the toilet or on your underwear.

Although brown spotting or even a little red blood present in early pregnancy is not uncommon, your doctor may want to examine you to see if your cervix is still tightly closed or if it is dilating, if your level of HCG (human chorionic gonadotropin) is increasing as it should (doubling about every forty-eight hours in the early weeks of pregnancy), and if a fetal sac can be seen in the uterus (in order to rule out an ectopic pregnancy) and the baby's heartbeat can be detected, both on ultrasound.[1]

Most often early bleeding stems from a benign source, such as:

1. Blood shed from the uterine wall when the embryo implants.

2. Breakthrough bleeding, when not quite enough pregnancy hormones are yet in your system to completely curtail menstruation.[2]

3. A sensitive cervix. During pregnancy your cervix may become irritated from even a careful medical exam or from getting gently bumped during intercourse.

Bright red blood together with cramps, or brown spotting that progresses to the flowing of bright red blood and is accompanied by increasingly heavy cramping, may be the beginning of a miscarriage. Miscarriage almost always happens because something is wrong with the pregnancy that is not preventable. Pregnancy loss is not caused by exercise, sex, work,[3] or anger or ambivalence about being pregnant.

Spotting or staining later in pregnancy can also be caused by an irritated cervix, but a condition called *placenta previa* is most often the cause of painless bleeding in your last trimester.[4] Sometimes the placenta lies low rather than on the side of the uterus, either partially or completely covering your cervix. Bleeding occurs as it pulls away when the cervix dilates even slightly.[5]

Abruptio placentae is a condition in which the placenta separates from the uterine wall before birth. The symptoms of abruptio placentae include bleeding and abdominal pain, both of which can be severe depending on the size of the area that has torn away.[6]

CONTRACTIONS

Contractions are normal throughout pregnancy,[7] however, when they become frequent or regular, they may be a symptom of preterm labor. Having five or more in an hour,[8] or contractions that occur regularly—coming every ten minutes, for example—are warning signs.[9]

Contractions can be painless, making them harder to detect. Thus even though physicians are not sure these painless contractions are precursors to preterm labor,[10] some recommend that you familiarize yourself with the pattern of contractions you normally experience in a day by checking for them for at least thirty minutes both morning and evening.[11]

Lying on your side, gently press your fingertips into your uterus. If you are having contractions, you will feel it alternating from soft and relaxed, to tensing up and becoming firm. Contractions are timed from the beginning of one to the beginning of the next.

By tuning into your body, you will be able to identify a baseline against which to compare changes in frequency of contractions, as well as any of the other signs associated with preterm labor. These include:[12]

1. Leaking or gushing water from your vagina.

2. Vaginal discharge that becomes heavier, mucusy, brownish, pinkish, or streaked with blood.

3. A feeling of pressure in your pelvis or groin.

4. Abdominal cramping.

5. A constant, dull ache in your lower back.

Do the following if you have regular contractions, experience five or more in an hour, or have any of the symptoms listed above:[13]

1. Urinate.

2. Lie down on your left side for sixty minutes.

3. Hydrate your system with three to four glasses of water or juice.

4. Feel your uterus and focus your attention on your contractions.

Call your doctor immediately if you experience any of the following during the next hour:[14]

1. The frequency of your contractions remains at five or more per hour.

2. Your contractions continue to occur regularly.

3. Any of your symptoms *worsen* at any point within that hour.

If they stop, but *return* after sixty minutes, call your physician.[15] If they go away completely, take it easy and avoid whatever activity may have triggered this episode. Speak with your doctor about your symptoms at your next appointment[16] or phone now if that's more comfortable for you than waiting.

LACK OF FETAL MOVEMENT

Your baby's movement may become easier to track toward the end of your sixth month, when his or her activity becomes stronger and more consistent than earlier.[17] At some point in late pregnancy your doctor may have you do "kick counts", where you note how long it takes for the baby to make ten movements at a regular time each day.

The baby's level of activity may change even from day to day, sometimes vigorous and seemingly nonstop, other times quiet and restful. Over time, you will develop a sense for the range of what feels normal. Keep in mind that the sleep cycle for most babies runs twenty to forty minutes,[18] and that you will probably find your baby is quieter when you're most active. However, if his or her movement reduces outside of that norm, or stops completely for longer than you've noticed before, call your doctor to discuss whether this might indicate a problem.

HEADACHES

Headaches that are unremitting or severe, along with sudden swelling, particularly facial swelling, and a rapid weight gain of more than 1 pound per day beyond the sixth month may be signs of pregnancy-induced hypertension,[19] also called preeclampsia or toxemia. Midlife women may be more susceptible, as are women of any age with their first baby.[20] This is especially so if high blood pressure is a preexisting condition, but most women who develop hypertension while pregnant have never had any such prior problem.[21] Call your doctor if you experience any of the above symptoms.

Other signs of potential problems in pregnancy that should lead you to call your doctor include:[22]

1. Vision becomes blurred, you see spots or flashes of light.

2. Abdominal pain concentrated in the upper right area.

3. Constant vomiting.

4. Fever, chills.

5. Gushing or leaking fluid from your vagina (more watery than vaginal discharge).

Appendix B

Basic Food Guide: Preconception-Pregnancy-Nursing

You are adding about 100 calories per day to your preconception diet for the first trimester, and about 300 (total) more daily for your second and third. If you nurse, you'll add an additional 200 per day after your baby is born, for a combined 500 calories daily over your *pre*pregnancy intake to meet the extra caloric demands of breastfeeding.[1] You'll want to incorporate one additional protein serving[2] and one additional calcium-rich food serving[3] daily over your pregnancy requirements into your nursing diet.

Amounts vary depending on your prepregnancy weight and your level of physical activity.[4] Consult your doctor or a registered dietitian with any questions you may have about individualizing your diet.

Food Summary[5]

PROTEIN FOODS	SERVINGS PER DAY
Preconception	2–3
Pregnancy	at least 3
Nursing	at least 4

CALCIUM-RICH FOODS	SERVINGS PER DAY
Preconception	2–3
Pregnancy	at least 3
Nursing	at least 4

FRUITS	SERVINGS PER DAY
Preconception	2–4
Pregnancy	at least 2
Nursing	at least 2

VEGETABLES	SERVINGS PER DAY
Preconception	3–5
Pregnancy	at least 3
Nursing	at least 3

GRAINS, BREADS AND CEREALS	SERVINGS PER DAY
Preconception	6–11
Pregnancy	at least 7
Nursing	at least 7

FLUIDS	8-ounce glass
Preconception	at least 6
Pregnancy	6–8
Nursing	at least 8

Fats: Limit to no more than 30 percent of daily calorie total.

Portion sizes equal to one serving:[6]

Protein Foods
Meat, poultry, fish—2 ounces
Eggs—2
Nuts—½ cup
Nut butters—¼ cup
Beans—1 cup cooked

Calcium-rich foods
Milk—1 cup
Cheese—1½ ounces
Cheese spread—4 tablespoons
Yogurt—1 cup
Cottage cheese—1⅓ cups
Broccoli—2 cups
Canned salmon with bones—3 ounces

Fruits and vegetables
Apple—1 medium
Orange—1 medium
Banana—1 medium
Strawberries—¾ cup
Cantaloupe—½ medium
Orange juice—4 ounces
Tomato juice—12 ounces
Raw, leafy vegetables—1 cup
Cauliflower, carrots, etc.—½ cup cooked or raw

Grains, bread and cereals
Bread—1 slice
Cereal: Hot—½ cup cooked
   Cold—1 ounce (¾–1½ cups)
Rice—½ cup cooked
Pasta—½ cup cooked
Crackers—4
Waffle—1 medium

Muffin—1 small
Bagel—1 small or ½ large
Tortilla—1
Wheat germ—1 tablespoon

Fluids
Water
Water-based liquids: Juices
                     Decaffeinated coffee
                     Decaffeinated tea

Nutrient-rich food sources[7]
Folate (folic acid)–rich foods
Fruits
Bananas
Orange juice
Grapefruit juice
Oranges
Cantaloupe
Watermelon
Avocados

Vegetables
Tomatoes
Cauliflower
Brussels sprouts
Broccoli
Green, leafy vegetables
Deep yellow vegetables

Iron-rich foods
Beef
Eggs
Dried fruit
Enriched cereals

Vegetables
Spinach
Broccoli
Brussels sprouts
Dark green lettuces

Calcium-rich foods
Milk
Milk products
Salmon with bones
Sardines with bones
Broccoli

Notes

SUPPLEMENTS

Preconception: Multivitamin that includes folic acid or an individual supplement. The current recommended dosage by the United States Center for Disease Control and Prevention for women in their childbearing years is 400 micrograms daily.[8] However, amounts may vary from source to source,[9] and are also periodically updated. Speak with your doctor for his or her best recommendation.

Pregnancy: The current recommendation for folic acid supplementation during pregnancy is also 400 micrograms daily[10] through at least your sixth week of pregnancy. The American College of Obstetricians and Gynecologists suggests supplementing during the first three months.[11] To ensure your increased iron needs are met, your doctor may suggest iron supplements or prenatal vitamins. Some women also have trouble taking in adequate calcium in their diets. Consult with your doctor about supplementing your iron or calcium intake during pregnancy.

ASPARTAME

The effects of this artificial sweetener, often marketed under the name NutraSweet, have not been researched in pregnant women. However, this substance has been widely studied otherwise since the early 1980s. Given the thorough knowledge of the way it works in the body, it is not thought to be harmful during pregnancy.[12]

SACCHARIN

Also an artificial sweetener, saccharin has been found to cause cancer in animal studies and to remain in the tissues. Nevertheless, it is unclear whether its use would actually harm a fetus. To be on the safe side, a limit of one to two packets per day is suggested.[13]

RAW FOODS

To safeguard against food-borne teratogens and against becoming ill from foods at this time when you're wanting to maintain your health at its best, during either the immediate preconception period and pregnancy, *don't eat:*

Raw fish or undercooked fish. May contain tapeworms or roundworms.

Raw or undercooked meats. May harbor the parasite causing toxoplasmosis.

Undercooked poultry. Salmonella, Escherichia coli.

Raw milk (unpasteurized). Salmonella, toxoplasmosis, listeriosis.

Raw or undercooked eggs. Salmonella, Escherichia coli.[14]

References

Introduction

1   Stephanie J. Ventura, AM, Joyce A. Martin, MPH, T.J. Matthews, MS, Sally C. Clarke, MA. "Advance Report of Final Natality Statistics, 1994." *Monthly Vital Statistics Report.* Hyattsville, Md.: National Center for Health Statistics. June 24, 1996; vol. 44, no. 11 supplement, p. 31.

2   Ibid., p. 29.

3   Gopal K. Singh, PhD, T.J. Matthews, MS, Sally C. Clarke, Trina Yannicos, and Betty L. Smith, Division of Vital Statistics. "Annual Summary of Birth, Marriages, Divorces and Deaths United States, 1994." *Monthly Vital Statistics Report.* Hyattsville, Md.: National Center for Health Statistics. October 23, 1995; vol. 43, no. 13, p. 17, table 7.

Chapter One: Before You Conceive

1   Daniel Navot, Paul A. Bergh, Mary Anne Williams, G. John Garrisi, Ida Guzman, Benjamin Sandler, Lawrence Grunfield. "Poor Oocyte Quality Rather Than Implantation Failure as a Cause of Age-Related

Decline in Female Fertility." *Lancet* vol. 337 (June 8, 1991): 1376, 1377. "Declining fertility: egg or uterus? Editorial." *Lancet* vol. 338 (August 3, 1991): 286.

2   William D. Mosher, PhD, William F. Pratt, PhD. "Fecundity and Infertility in the United States, 1965–88." *Advance Data*. Vital and Health Statistics. Hyattsville, Md: National Center for Health Statistics. December 4, 1990; no. 192, p. 3, table 1. Kathleen Diamond, PhD. *Motherhood After Miscarriage*. Holbrook, Ma.: Bob Adams, Inc., 1991, 215. Interview, Samuel Wood, MD, PhD, 3/21/94.

3   Interview. Samuel Wood, MD, PhD, 5/20/96. Wood, 3/21/94.

4   FIVNAT. C. Piette, J. de Mouzon, A. Bachelot, A. Spira. "In-Vitro Fertilization: Influence of Women's Age on Pregnancy Rates." *Human Reproduction* vol. 5, no. 1 (1990): 56. Santiago L. Padilla, MD, Jairo E. Garcia, MD. "Effect of Maternal Age and Number of In Vitro Fertilization Procedures on Pregnancy Outcome." *Fertility and Sterility* vol. 52, no. 2 (August 1989): 273. MJ Faddy, RG Gosden, A. Gougeon, Sandra J. Richardson, JF Nelson. "Accelerated Disappearance of Ovarian Follicles in Mid-Life: Implications for Forecasting Menopause." *Human Reproduction* vol. 7, no. 10 (1992): 1342, 1345.

5   Interview. Carol Harter, MD. 2/28/94.

6   Personal communication. Samuel Wood, MD, PhD. 12/23/96.

7   Stephanie J. Ventura, AM, Joyce A. Martin, MPH, T.J. Matthews, MS, Sally C. Clarke, MD. "Advance Report of Final Natality Statistics, 1994." *Monthly Vital Statistics Report*. Hyattsville, Md.: National Center for Health Statistics. June 24, 1996; vol. 44, no. 11 supplement, p. 29.

8   American College of Obstetricians and Gynecologists. (ACOG). *Planning for Pregnancy, Birth and Beyond*. Second edition. New York: Dutton, New York. 1996, p. 13.

9   Allen J. Wilcox, MD, PhD, Clarice R. Weinberg, PhD, Donna R. Baird, PhD. "Timing of Sexual Intercourse in Relation to Ovulation." *New England Journal of Medicine* vol. 333, no. 23 (December 7, 1995): 1520.

10   Margie Profet. *Protecting Your Baby-to-Be: Preventing Birth Defects in the First Trimester*. Reading, Mass: Addison-Wesley, 1995, p. 1–3.

11   Mosher, Pratt, "Fecundity and Infertility in the United States," 1965–88, p. 3, table 1. Ventura et al., "Advance Report of Final Natality Statistics, 1994," p. 5.

12 California Teratogen Information Service and Clinical Research Program. UCSD Medical Center, University of California, San Diego. Teratogen Information Specialist. 1/6/94.

13 Personal communication. Janice Baker, RD, Certified Diabetes Educator. 11/4/96.

14 Niels H. Lauersen, MD, PhD, Colette Bouchez. *Getting Pregnant: What Couples Need to Know Right Now*. New York: Fawcett Columbine, 1991, p. 7.

15 Consumer Reports Books. Ovulation Prediction Test Kits for Home Use. *Complete Drug Reference*. 1995 edition. Yonkers, NY: Consumers Union of United States, p. 1266.

16 Wilcox, et al., "Timing of Sexual Intercourse in Relation to Ovulation," p. 1520.

17 Consumer Reports Books, "Ovulation Prediction Test Kits for Home Use," p. 1266.

18 Lauersen, Bouchez, *Getting Pregnant*, p. 201.

19 Wilcox, et al. "Timing of Sexual Intercourse in Relation to Ovulation," p. 1517, 1518.

20 Personal communication. Samuel Wood, MD, PhD. 12/10/96.

21 Wilcox, et al., "Timing of Sexual Intercourse in Relation to Ovulation," p. 1519, figure 2, p. 1520, figure 3.

22 Boston Women's Health Book Collective. *The New Our Bodies, Ourselves*. New York: Simon and Schuster, 1992; p. 276.

23 Peggy Robin. *How to Be a Successful Fertility Patient*. New York: William Morrow, 1993, p. 37.

24 Boston Women's Health Book Collective, *The New Our Bodies, Ourselves*, p. 280.

25 ACOG, *Planning for Pregnancy, Birth and Beyond*, p. 7.

26 *Mosby Medical Encyclopedia*. Revised edition. New York: Plume, 1992, p. 510.

27 Boston's Women's Health Book Collective, *The New Our Bodies, Ourselves*, p. 248.

28 ACOG. *Planning for Pregnancy, Birth and Beyond*, pp. 5, 152, 156, 161. *Mosby*, p. 40. Sheila Kitzinger. *The Complete Book of Pregnancy and*

Childbirth. New York: Knopf, 1986, p. 123. Phyllis Kernoff Mansfield, *Pregnancy for Older Women: Assessing the Medical Risks.* New York: Praeger, 1986, p. 93, 94.

29 ACOG, *Planning for Pregnancy, Birth and Beyond,* p. 149. *Mosby,* p. 394.

30 ACOG, *Planning for Pregnancy, Birth and Beyond,* p. 152.

31 *Mosby,* p. 244.

32 ACOG, *Planning for Pregnancy, Birth and Beyond,* p. 156.

33 Ibid., p. 155.

34 Ibid.

35 *Mosby,* p. 510.

36 Wood, 5/20/96.

37 Wood, 12/23/96. ACOG, *Planning for Pregnancy, Birth and Beyond,* p. 20.

38 Robin, *How to Be a Successful Fertility Patient,* pp. 157, 158.

39 *Mosby,* p. 285.

40 Mansfield, *Pregnancy for Older Women,* pp. 95, 96.

41 Kathryn Schrotenboer-Cox, ob/gyn and Joan Solomon Weiss. *Pregnancy over 35.* New York: Ballantine Books. 1985, p. 94.

42 Boston Women's Health Book Collective, *The New Our Bodies, Ourselves,* pp. 583, 584.

43 National Cancer Institute, National Institute of Child Health and Human Development, National Institutes of Health. *DES DAUGHTERS: Women Born Between 1938 and 1971 Who Were Exposed to DES Before Birth.* Pamphlet, p. 4.

44 Ibid., cover.

45 Ibid., pp. 23–25.

46 Ibid., p. 15.

47 Ibid., pp. 15, 17, 19.

48 ACOG, *Planning for Pregnancy, Birth and Beyond,* p. 13.

49 Ibid.

50 *Mosby*, pp. 167, 374, 349, 744. ACOG, *Planning for Pregnancy, Birth and Beyond*, p. 184.

51 "Foodborne Illness: Role of Home Food Handling Practices." *Food Technology* vol. 49, no. 4 (April 1995): 124. Reprinted from the American Council on Science and Health (ACSH). New York.

52 Kaiser Permanente. *Having a Healthy, Happy Baby. Prenatal Infosheet #1.* Health Education. Obstetrics and Gynecology, San Diego, 6/95, p. 9.

53 Personal communication. Kathryn Baker. California State Office of AIDS. 10/10/96.

54 ACOG, *Planning for Pregnancy, Birth and Beyond*, p. 13.

55 *Mosby*, p. 688.

56 Ibid.

57 ACOG, *Planning for Pregnancy, Birth and Beyond*, p. 13.

58 *Mosby*, p. 688.

59 Ibid., p. 371

60 ACOG, *Planning for Pregnancy, Birth and Beyond*, p. 194.

61 Ibid.

62 Ibid.

63 *Mosby*, p. 490.

64 ACOG, *Planning for Pregnancy, Birth and Beyond*, p. 190.

65 *Mosby*, p. 489.

66 Ibid., p. 518.

67 ACOG, *Planning for Pregnancy, Birth and Beyond*, p. 192.

68 Ibid., p. 190.

69 Ibid.

70 *Mosby*, p. 618.

71 Ibid.

72 ACOG, *Planning for Pregnancy, Birth and Beyond*, p. 13.

73 Ibid., p. 71.

74   Ibid., pp. 69, 70.

75   Ibid., p. 67.

76   Profet, *Protecting Your Baby-to-Be*, pp. 1–3, 172.

77   ACOG. *Planning for Pregnancy, Birth and Beyond*, pp. 118, 119. "Dietary Guidelines Modified from the United States Department of Agriculture and United States Department of Health and Human Services." Kaiser Permanente. *Eating for Two, Nutrition for Pregnancy and Breast Feeding*. Health Education Pamphlet. Southern California region. 8/82. Personal communication. Janice Baker, RD, Certified Diabetes Educator. 5/15/97.

78   ACOG, *Planning for Pregnancy, Birth and Beyond*, p. 7.

79   United States Department of Health and Human Services. (DHHS) "Recommendations for the Use of Folic Acid to Reduce the Number of Cases of Spina Bifida and Other Neural Tube Defects." *Center for Disease Control Morbidity and Mortality Weekly Report* vol. 41, no. rr-14 (September 11, 1992): 1.

80   Kaiser Permanente, *Eating for Two*.

81   United Stated DHHS, "Recommendations for the Use of Folic Acid," p. 5.

82   Personal communication. Richard Olney, MD. Medical epidermiologist, Center for Disease Control and Prevention. 12/23/96.

83   Profet, *Protecting Your Baby-to-Be*, p. 172.

84   ACOG, *Planning for Pregnancy, Birth and Beyond*, p. 76.

85   Baker, 11/4/96.

86   Kitzinger, *Complete Book of Pregnancy*, p. 87.

87   Baker, 11/4/96.

88   Kaiser Permanente, *Eating for Two*. Boston Women's Health Book Collective, *The New Our bodies, Ourselves*, p. 39.

89   Kaiser Permanente, *Eating for Two*.

90   Personal communication. Janice Baker, RD, Certified Diabetes Educator. 9/9/96.

91   William N. Spellacy, MD, Stephen J. Miller, MD, Ann Winegar, MS. "Pregnancy after 40 Years of Age." *Obstetrics and Gynecology* vol. 68, no. 4 (October 1986): 454.

92 Gertrud S. Berkowitz, PhD, Mary Louise Skovron, DrPh, Robert H. Lapinski, PhD, Richard L. Berkowitz, MD. "Delayed Childbearing and the Outcome of Pregnancy." *New England Journal of Medicine* vol. 322, no. 10 (March 8, 1990): 661.

93 Lauersen, Bouchez, *Getting Pregnant*, pp. 145, 147.

94 Wood, 5/20/96.

95 Gary M. Shaw, DrPh, Ellen M. Velie, MPH, Donna Schaffer, MPH, RD. "Risk of Neural Tube Defect–Affected Pregnancies Among Obese Women." *Journal of the American Medical Association* vol. 275, no. 14 (April 10, 1996): 1093. Martha M. Werler, ScD, Carol Louik, ScD, Samuel Shapiro, MD, FRCPE, Allen A. Mitchell, MD. "Prepregnant Weight in Relation to Risk of Neural Tube Defects." *Journal of the American Medical Association* vol. 275, no. 14 (April 10, 1996): 1089.

96 Richard L. Naeye. "Maternal Body Weight and Pregnancy Outcome." *American Journal of Clinical Nutrition* vol. 52, (1990) 273.

97 Wood, 5/20/96.

98 California Teratogen Information Service and Clinical Research Program. Teratogen Information Specialist. 5/8/96.

99 Ibid.

100 Wood, 12/10/96.

101 Elizabeth G. Raymond, Sven Cnattingius, John L. Kiely. "Effects of Maternal Age, Parity, and Smoking on the Risk of Stillbirth." *British Journal of Obstetrics and Gynaecology* vol. 101 (April 1994): 302.

102 Ventura, et al. "Advance Report of Final Natality Statistics, 1994," pp. 2, 12.

103 Ibid., p. 12.

104 National Institutes of Health, as cited by Lauersen, Bouchez, *Getting Pregnant*, p. 164.

105 Dairy Council of California. *Pregnancy: A Special Time for Nutrition and Good Health.* 1993, p. 8.

106 Lauersen, Bouchez, *Getting Pregnant*, p. 164.

107 Profet, *Protecting Your Baby-to-Be*, pp. 175, 176.

108 Lori L. Altshuler, MD, Lee Cohen, MD, Martin P. Szuba, MD, Vivien K. Burt, MD, PhD, Michael Gitlin, MD, Jim Mintz, PhD. "Pharmaco-

logic Management of Psychiatric Illness During Pregnancy: Dilemmas and Guidelines." *American Journal of Psychiatry* vol. 153, no. 5 (May 1996): 592, 602.

109 Ibid., p. 599.

110 California Teratogen Information Service and Clinical Research Program. Teratogen Information Specialist, 5/8/96.

111 Ibid.

112 Personal communication, Glenda Spivey, MS. President of OTIS, Organization of Teratogen Information Specialists. 4/22/97. Personal communication. Lynn Martinez, Program Manager, Pregnancy Risk Line, Utah State Department of Health and Past President of OTIS. 5/1/97.

113 California Teratogen Information Service and Clinical Research Program. Teratogen Information Specialist, 5/8/96.

114 Kaiser Permanente, *Having a Healthy, Happy Baby*, p. 9.

115 Ibid.

116 Personal communication. Larry Smarr, President, Physician Insurers Association of America. 8/29/96, 5/19/97.

117 B. Neugarten. "Social Clocks." 1972. As cited by Julia C. Berryman, Bsc, PhD, C.Psychol, AFBPsS, Kate Windridge, Bsc, PhD. "Having a Baby After 40: A Preliminary Investigation of Women's Experience of Pregnancy." *Journal of Reproductive and Infant Psychology* vol. 9, (1991) 3.

118 Vital Statistics of the United States. United States Department of Health and Human Services. Public Health Service. Hyattsville, Md; 1988; vol. I—*Natality*. p. 7. Ventura, et al., "Advance Report of Final Natality Statistics, 1994," p. 31.

119 Phyllis Kernoff Mansfield, PhD, William McCool, RN, CNM, MS. "Toward a Better Understanding of the 'Advanced Maternal Age' Factor." *Health Care for Women International* vol. 10 (1989): 408.

120 Stephanie J. Ventura, AM, Joyce A. Martin, MPH, Selma M. Taffel, T.J. Matthews, MS, Sally C. Clarke. "Advance Report of Final Natality Statistics, 1993." *Monthly Vital Statistics Report*. Hyattsville, Md. National Center for Health Statistics. September 21, 1995; vol. 44, no. 3 supplement, p. 5. Ventura, et al., "Advance Report of Final Natality Statistics, 1994," pp. 5, 29.

121 Robert Kominski, Andrea Adams. "Educational Attainment in the United States: March 1993 and 1992." *Current Population Reports, Popu-*

lation Characteristics. United States Department of Commerce Bureau of the Census. May 1994; p20–476, p. VII, XI.

122 Ventura, et al. "Advance Report of Final Natality Statistics, 1994," p. 10.

123 Raymond, et al. "Effects of Maternal Age, Parity and Smoking on the Risk of Stillbirth," p. 303.

124 Christine L. Roberts, Charles S. Algert, Lyn M. March. "Delayed Childbearing—Are There Any Risks?" *Medical Journal of Australia* vol. 160 (May 2, 1994): 539.

125 Christopher O'Reilly-Green, MD, Wayne R. Cohen, MD. "Pregnancy in Women Aged 40 and Older." *Obstetrics and Gynecology Clinics of North America:* vol. 20, no. 2 (June 1993) 327.

126 Ventura, et al. "Advance Report of Final Natality Statistics, 1993," pp. 10, 11.

127 Michael Prysak, PhD, MD, Robert P. Lorenz, MD, Anne Kisly. "Pregnancy Outcome in Nulliparous Women 35 Years and Older." *Obstetrics and Gynecology* vol. 85, no. 1 (January 1995). Spellacy, et al., "Pregnancy After 40 Years of Age," p. 452. MJ Brassil, MJ Turner, DM Egan, DW MacDonald. "Obstetric Outcome in First-Time Mothers Aged 40 Years and Over." *European Journal of Obstetrics, Gynecology and Reproductive Biology* vol. 25 (1987): 115, 120. The two following studies conclude only that older mothers experience higher rates of medical problems during their pregnancies, and yet their babies generally remain unaffected and healthy. Berkowitz, et al., "Delayed Childbearing and the Outcome of Pregnancy," pp. 659, 662, 663. O'Reilly-Green, Cohen. "Pregnancy in Women Aged 40 and Older," p. 327.

128 Wood, 5/20/96.

129 O'Reilly-Green, Cohen. "Pregnancy in Women Aged 40 and Older," pp. 319, 320. Brassil, et al. "Obstetric Outcome in First-Time Mothers Aged 40 Years and Over," p. 119. VickiLee Edge, MD, Russell K. Laros, Jr., MD. "Pregnancy Outcome in Nulliparous Women Aged 35 or Older." *American Journal of Obstetrics and Gynecology* vol. 168, no. 6, part 1 (June 1993): 1881, 1883. Diane Gordon, MS, MPH, John Milberg, MPH, Janet Daling, PhD, Durlin Hickok, MD, MPH. "Advanced Maternal Age as a Risk Factor for Cesarean Delivery." *Obstetrics and Gynecology* vol. 77, no. 4 (April 1991) 493, 496. Berkowitz, et al. "Delayed Childbearing and the Outcome of Pregnancy," p. 662.

130 Edge, Laros. "Pregnancy Outcome in Nulliparous Women Aged 35 or Older," pp. 1881, 1883. Gordon, et al., "Advanced Maternal Age as a Risk Factor for Cesarean Delivery," p. 493. Method A. Duchon, MD, Kevin L. Muise, MD. "Pregnancy After Age 35." *Female Patient* vol. 18 (June 1993): 71. O'Reilly-Green, Cohen. "Pregnancy in Women Aged 40 and Older," p. 320. Brassil, et al., "Obstetric Outcome in First-Time Mothers Aged 40 Years and Over," p. 119. Berkowitz, et al., "Delayed Childbearing and the Outcome of Pregnancy," p. 662.

131 Joseph A. Adashek, MD, Alan M. Peaceman, MD, Jose A. Lopez-Zena, MD, John P. Minogue, DMin, Michael L. Socol, MD. "Factors Contributing to the Increased Cesarean Birth Rate in Older Parturient Women." *American Journal of Obstetrics and Gynecology* vol. 169, no. 4 (1993): 936, 939.

132 Brassil, et al., "Obstetric Outcome in First-Time Mothers Aged 40 Years and Over," p. 119.

133 Beth Weinhouse. "Is There a Right Time to Have a Baby?" *Glamour.* May 1994, p. 285.

134 Allen T. Bombard, MD, Robert W. Naef III, MD. "Reproductive Genetics for Couples Older Than 40 Years of Age." *Obstetrics and Gynecology Clinics of North America* vol. 20, no. 2 (June 1993): 282.

135 Edge, Laros. "Pregnancy Outcome in Nulliparous Women Aged 35 or Older," p. 1881. Berkowitz, et al., "Delayed Childbearing and the Outcome of Pregnancy," pp. 659, 663.

136 Bombard, Naef. "Reproductive Genetics for Couples Older Than 40 Years of Age," p. 282.

Chapter Two: A Preconception ShortCut

1   Interview. Samuel Wood, MD, PhD. 5/20/96. James P. Toner, MD, PhD, Jill Taylor Flood, MD. "Fertility After the Age of 40." *Obstetrics and Gynecology Clinics of North America* vol. 20, no. 2 (June 1993): 263–66.

2   Niels H. Lauersen, MD, PhD, Collette Bouchez. *Getting Pregnant: What Couples Need to Know Right Now.* New York: Fawcett Columbine 1991, p. 7.

3   Wood, 5/20/96.

4   Ibid. Toner, Flood. "Fertility After the Age of 40," pp. 263–66.

5   Interview. Carol Harter, MD. 2/28/94. Interview. Samuel Wood, MD,
     PhD. 3/21/94. Serono Symposia, USA. *Infertility over 35*. Patient infor-
     mation pamphlet. Serono Laboratories, Norwell, Mass. 9/93; inside
     cover.

6   Harter, 2/28/94. Interview. William Hummel, MD. 2/23/94.

Chapter Three: Prenatal Testing: Embracing Your Pregnancy, Finally

1   AT Bombard, MD, RW Naef III, MD. "Reproductive Genetics for
     Couples Older Than 40 Years of Age." *Obstetrics and Gynecology Clin-
     ics of North America* vol. 20, no. 2 (1993) 282. Kaiser Permanente. *Sum-
     mary of Prenatal Diagnosis Procedures*. Health education. Southern
     California region, 9/95. American College of Obstetricians and Gyne-
     cologists (ACOG), *Planning for Pregnancy, Birth and Beyond*. Second
     edition. New York: Dutton, 1996, p. 84.

2   Kaiser Permanente. *Amniocentesis for Prenatal Diagnosis*. Health educa-
     tion pamphlet. Southern California region, May 1988; p. 7. ACOG,
     Planning for Pregnancy, Birth and Beyond, p. 79.

3   Personal communication. Gloria Anne Sanchez-Araiza, MS, MPH,
     Certified Genetics Counselor, 12/13/96.

4   Bombard, Naef, "Reproductive Genetics for Couples Older Than 40,"
     p. 282.

5   Kaiser Permanente, *Summary of Prenatal Diagnosis Procedures*.

6   Bombard, Naef, "Reproductive Genetics for Couples Older Than 40,"
     p. 282.

7   Kaiser Permanente, *Summary of Prenatal Diagnosis Procedures*.

8   United States Department of Health and Human Services (DHHS).
     "Chorionic Villus Sampling and Amniocentesis: Recommendations
     for Prenatal Counseling." *Center for Disease Control Morbidity and Mor-
     tality Weekly Report* vol. 44, no. RR-9, (July 21, 1995): 4.

9   Kathleen Diamond, PhD. *Motherhood After Miscarriage*. Holbrook, Mass.: Bob Adams, Inc., 1991, pp. 100, 101.

10 ACOG, *Planning for Pregnancy, Birth and Beyond*, p. 81.

11 *The Mosby Medical Encyclopedia*. Revised edition. New York: Plume, 1992, p. 721.

12 ACOG, *Planning for Pregnancy, Birth and Beyond*, p. 75.

13 Ibid., pp. 74, 75.

14 Ibid., pp. 79, 81, 82.

15 Ibid., p. 84.

16 Kaiser Permanente, *Summary of Prenatal Diagnosis Procedures*.

17 Family Planning Associates. San Diego. 11/13/96.

18 Laird G. Jackson, MD, Maurice J. Mahoney, MD, Michael T. Mennuti, MD, Joe Leigh Simpson, MD (moderator). "Weighing the Advantages CVS Confers." *Contemporary Ob/Gyn* (January 1993): 124.

19 ACOG, *Planning for Pregnancy, Birth and Beyond*, p. 52.

20 Bruce Jancin. "Data Suggest CVS Is Safer Than Thought." Printed in *Ob. Gyn News*, April 1, 1996, p. 37.

21 Ibid., p. 38. Simpson, et al. "Weighing the Advantages CVS Confers," p. 124. Larry Cousins, MD, Kathy O'Hanlon-Carder, MS, Certified Genetics Counselor, Barbara Dixson, RN, MN, Certified Genetics Counselor. "Chorionic Villus Sampling or Early Amniocentesis for Prenatal Diagnosis?" *Sharp Perinatal Newsletter*. Staff newsletter, Sharp Hospital, San Diego. August 11, 1993, p. 3.

22 Personal Communication. Gloria Anne Sanchez-Araiza, MS, MPH, Certified Genetics Counselor, 11/24/97.

23 Simpson, et al., "Weighing the Advantages CVS Confers," p. 124.

24 California Department of Health Services—Genetic Disease Branch (DHS—GDB). *Prenatal Diagnosis Center Standards and Definitions*. Berkeley, Calif., 1997.

25 Personal communication. Linda Foley, MS. California Department of Health Services—Genetic Disease Branch. Berkeley, Calif. 4/8/97.

26 Personal communication. Sara Goldman, MPH. California Department of Health Services—Genetic Disease Branch. Berkeley, Calif. 4/9/97.

27 Personal communication. Paula Weber, RN, BSN, Genetics Nurse. 12/16/96.

28 Personal communication. Barbara Dixson, RN, MSN, Certified Genetics Counselor. 12/16/96.

29 Weber, 12/16/96.

30 Family Planning Associates. 11/13/96, 9/9/96.

31 ACOG, *Planning for Pregnancy, Birth and Beyond*, p. 27. *Mosby*, p. 173.

32 ACOG, *Amniocentesis and Chorionic Villus Sampling*, Patient education pamphlet. June 1995; p. 6. ACOG, *Planning for Pregnancy, Birth and Beyond*, p. 84.

33 ACOG, *Planning for Pregnancy, Birth and Beyond*, p. 84.

34 United States DHHS. "Chorionic Villus Sampling and Amniocentesis: Recommendations," p. 4. Kaiser Permanente, *Summary of Prenatal Diagnosis Procedures*.

35 Maria Martins, MD, Anthony Johnson, DO. "Does Chorionic Villus Sampling Cause Limb Defects?" Section of Genetics, Pennsylvania Hospital, Philadelphia. *Genetics and Teratology* vol. 2, no. 1 (June 1993): 1, 2. Simpson, et al., "Weighing the Advantages CVS Confers," pp. 112, 114.

36 Ibid. Mitchel L. Zoler. "Persistent Concerns about Safety Hinder Wider Use of Chorionic Villus Sampling." Printed in *Ob.Gyn. News* vol. 29, no. 5 (March 1, 1994): 9.

37 Firth et al., "Severe Limb Abnormalities After Chorionic Villus Sampling at 56–66 Days' Gestation." *Lancet* 337 (1991): 762–3. Burton, et al., "Limb Abnormalities Associated with Chorionic Villus Sampling." *Obstetrics and Gynecology*, 79 (1992): 726–30. Cited in "Report of National Institute of Child Health and Human Development (NICHHD) on Chorionic Villus Sampling and Limb and Other Defects, October 20, 1992." *American Journal of Obstetrics and Gynecology* vol. 169, no. 1 (July 1993): 1, 2.

38 "Report of NICHHD Workshop," p. 1. Simpson, et al, "Weighing the Advantages CVS Confers," p. 122.

39 United States DHHS, "Chorionic Villus Sampling and Amniocentesis: Recommendations," pp. 4, 6, 7.

40 Ibid., pp. 6, 7.

41 Jancin, "Data Suggest CVS Is Safer Than Thought," p. 39.

42 Laird Jackson, as cited in United States DHHS, "Chorionic Villus Sampling and Amniocentesis: Recommendations," p. 2.

43 Martin, Johnson. "Does Chorionic Villus Sampling Cause Limb Defects?," p. 3. The American College of Obstetricians and Gyncologists. (AC06) Committee on Genetics. "Chorionic Villus Sampling." *Committee Opinion* no. 160 (October 1995): 2. Simpson, et al., "Weighing the Advantages CVS Confers," p. 124. Jancin, "Data Suggest CVS Is Safer Than Thought," pp. 38, 39. United States DHHS, "Chorionic Villus Sampling and Amniocentesis: Recommendations," p. 9. "Report of NICHHD Workshop," p. 3.

44 Jancin, "Data Suggest CVS Is Safer Than Thought," pp. 1, 38. Simpson, et al., "Weighing the Advantages CVS Confers," p. 124.

45 "Report of NICHHD Workshop," pp. 4, 5.

46 Jancin, "Data Suggest CVS Is Safer Than Thought," p. 38.

47 Ibid., p. 39. Martins, Johnson. "Does Chorionic Villus Sampling Cause Limb Defects?" p. 3.

48 Jancin, "Data Suggest CVS Is Safer Than Thought," p. 39. "Report of NICHHD Workshop," p. 5.

49 Jancin, "Data Suggest CVS Is Safer Than Thought," p. 39.

50 Ibid., p. 38.

51 Simpson, et al. "Weighing the Advantages CVS Confers," p. 114.

52 Burton, et al., "Limb Abnormalities Associated with Chorionic Villus Sampling," as cited in "Report of NICHHD Workshop," p. 2.

53 United States DHHS, "Chorionic Villus Sampling and Amniocentesis: Recommendations," p. 8. Cousins, et al., "Chorionic Villus Sampling or Early Amniocentesis," pp. 2, 3. Martins, Johnson. "Does Chorionic Villus Sampling Cause Limb Defects?" p. 3.

54 Martins, Johnson. "Does Chorionic Villus Sampling Cause Limb Defects?," p. 3. ACOG, "Chorionic Villus Sampling," p. 2.

55 Lauren Lynch, MD, as quoted in Zoler, "Persistent Concerns about Safety Hinder Wider Use," p. 9.

56 California DHHS—GDB, *Prenatal Diagnosis Center Standards and Definitions,* pp. 6, 7.

57 Goldman, 4/9/97.

58 California DHHS—GDB, *Prenatal Diagnosis Center Standards and Definitions*, pp. 6, 7.

59 Personal communication. Sara Goldman, MPH. California Department of Health Services—Genetic Disease Branch. Berkeley, Calif. 4/4/97.

60 United States DHHS, "Chorionic Villus Sampling and Amniocentesis: Recommendations," p. 2.

61 Jancin, "Data Suggest CVS Is Safer Than Thought," p. 39. Janis Grahm, *Your Pregnancy Companion.* New York: Pocket Books, 1991, p. 75.

62 United States DHHS, "Chorionic Villus Sampling and Amniocentesis: Recommendations," p. 4. Kaiser Permanente, *Summary of Prenatal Diagnosis Procedures.*

63 Kaiser Permanente, *Prenatal Diagnosis—Chorionic Villus Sampling (CVS).* Health education pamphlet. Southern California region. June 1989, p. 5.

64 Simpson, et al. "Weighing the Advantages CVS Confers," p. 109.

65 ACOG, *Amniocentesis and Chorionic Villus Sampling,* p. 6.

66 ACOG, *Pregnancy, Birth and Beyond,* p. 69.

67 Sanchez-Araiza, 12/13/96.

68 California DHS—GDB. *The California Alpha Fetoprotein Screening Program—Prenatal Screening Tests for Neural Tube and Other Birth Defects.* Pamphlet. Berkeley, Calif. January 1992, p. 2.

69 California DHS—GDB. *California Alpha Fetoprotein Screening Program,* p. 5.

70 ACOG, *Planning for Pregnancy, Birth and Beyond,* p. 81.

71 California DHS—GDB. *California Alpha Fetoprotein Screening Program,* p. 3.

72 Marnie L. MacDonald, MS, PhD, Roseanna M. Wagner, BS, R. Nathan Slotnick, MD, PhD. "Sensitivity and Specificity of Screening for Down Syndrome with Alpha Fetoprotein, HCG, Unconjugated Estriol, and Maternal Age." *Obstetrics and Gynecology* vol. 77, no. 1 (January 1991): 66, 67.

73 Personal communication. Mayland Arrington, Clinical Laboratory Scientist, Owner, Claydelle Clinical Laboratory. El Cajon, Calif. 5/6/97.

74 Jurgen Herrman, MD. "Triple-Marker Screening of Serum for Down's Syndrome." *New England Journal of Medicine* vol. 333, no. 10 (September 8, 1994): 681. California Department of Health Services—Genetic Disease Branch. *The Expanded AFP Test for Pregnant Women.* Pamphlet. Berkeley, Calif. 1995.

75 California DHS—GDB. *Prenatal Testing Choices for Women 35 Years and Older.* Pamphlet. Berkeley, Calif. 1995, p. 5.

76 Ernest B. Hook, MD. "Rates of Chromosome Abnormalities at Different Maternal Ages." *Obstetrics and Gynecology* vol. 58, no. 3 (September 1981): 283.

77 California DHS—GDB, *Prenatal Testing Choices for Women 35 Years and Older,* p. 6.

78 Personal communication. Robert J. Currier, PhD. Biostatistician, California Department of Health Services—Genetic Disease Branch. Berkeley, Calif. 11/14/96.

79 California DHS—GDB, *Prenatal Testing Choices for Women 35 Years and Older,* p. 6.

80 ACOG, *Planning for Pregnancy, Birth and Beyond,* pp. 79, 81, 82.

81 Weber, 12/16/96.

82 California DHS—GDB. *Prenatal Testing Choices for Women 35 Years and Older,* p. 6.

83 Ibid., p. 7.

84 ACOG, *Planning for Pregnancy, Birth and Beyond,* p. 82.

85 James E. Haddow, MD, Glenn E. Palomaki, BS, George J. Knight, PhD, George C. Cunningham, MD, Linda S. Lustig, MS, Patricia A. Boyd, MA. "Reducing the Need for Amniocentesis in Women 35 Years of Age or Older with Serum Markers for Screening." *New England Journal of Medicine* vol. 330, no. 16 (April 21, 1994): 1117. MacDonald, et al. "Sensitivity and Specificity of Screening for Down Syndrome," p. 68.

86 Dixson, 12/16/96.

87 California DHS—GDB. *Prenatal Testing Choices for Women 35 Years and Older,* p. 10.

88 Herrman, "Triple-Marker Screening of Serum for Down's Syndrome," p. 682.

89 J.R. Beekhuis, B.T.H.M. De Wolf, A. Mantingh, M.P. Heringa. "The Influence of Serum Screening on the Amniocentesis Rate in Women of Advanced Maternal Age." *Prenatal Diagnosis* vol. 14 (1994): 201.

90 Personal communication. George Cunningham, MD, MPH. Chief of the Genetic Disease Branch, California Department of Health Services. Berkeley, Calif. 7/14/97.

91 ACOG, *Planning for Pregnancy, Birth and Beyond*, p. 83.

92 *Mosby*, p. 802.

93 ACOG, *Planning for Pregnancy, Birth and Beyond*, p. 52.

94 Sanchez-Araiza, 12/13/96

Chapter Four: Fertility Treatment: When, Who, and What

1 William D. Mosher, PhD, William F. Pratt, PhD. "Fecundity and Infertility in the United States, 1965–88." *Advance Data.* Vital and Health Statistics. Hyattsville, Md.: National Center for Health Statistics. December 4, 1990; no. 192, p. 3, table 1.

2 Samuel Wood, MD, PhD. Interview. 5/11/94.

3 Ibid. Stephanie J. Ventura, AM, Joyce A. Martin, MPH, T.J. Matthews, MS, Sally C. Clarke, MA. "Advance Report of Final Natality Statistics, 1994." *Monthly Vital Statistics Report.* Hyattsville, Md.: National Center for Health Statistics. June 24, 1996; vol. 44, no. 11 supplement, p. 31.

4 M.J. Faddy, R.G. Gosden, A. Gougeon, Sandra J. Richardson, J.F. Nelson. "Accelerated Disappearance of Ovarian Follicles in Mid-Life: Implications for Forecasting Menopause." *Human Reproduction* vol. 7, no. 10 (1992): 1342.

5 Mosher, et al., "Fecundity and Infertility in the United States," p. 5.

6 Ibid., pp. 5, 6.

7   Interview. Samuel Wood, MD, PhD. 3/21/94.

8   Mosher, et al., "Fertility and Infertility in the United States," p. 1.

9   Wood, 3/21/94.

10 Wood, 5/11/94.

11 Interview. Carol Harter, MD. 2/28/94. Wood, 3/21/94. Serono Symposia, USA. *Infertility Over 35.* Patient information pamphlet. Serono Laboratories, Norwell, Mass. 9/93; inside cover.

12 Interview. William Hummel, MD. 2/23/94. Harter, 2/28/94.

13 Hummel, 2/23/94. Wood, 3/21/94.

14 Ibid. Wood, 5/11/94.

15 Wood, 3/21/94, 5/11/94.

16 Samuel Wood, MD, PhD. Notes.

17 Wood, 3/21/94.

18 Ibid.

19 Wood, 3/21/94, 5/11/94.

20 Wood, 3/21/94.

21 Wood, 3/21/94, 5/11/94.

22 Wood, notes.

23 William P. Hummel, MD, Mary G. Hammond, MD. "Infertility: The Evaluation of a Couple." *Obstetrics and Gynecology* (June 1989): 47.

24 Hummel, 2/23/94.

25 Serono Symposia, USA. *Insights into Infertility.* Patient information pamphlet. Serono Laboratories, Norwell, Mass. 4/93, p. 6.

26 Peggy Robin. *How to Be a Successful Fertility Patient.* New York: William Morrow, 1993, p. 130.

27 Serono Symposia, USA. *Insights into Infertility,* p. 5.

28 Wood, notes.

29 Robin, *How to Be a Successful Fertility Patient,* p. 123.

30 Personal communication. Samuel Wood, MD, PhD. 5/21/97.

31 Serono Symposia, USA. *Insights into Infertility,* p. 7.

32   Ibid., pp. 7, 8.

33   Ibid., p. 8.

34   Wood, notes.

35   Wood, 5/11/94.

36   Robin, *How to Be a Successful Fertility Patient*, pp. 125, 126.

37   Serono Symposia, USA. *Insights into Infertility*, p. 6.

38   Lynne S. Wilcox, MD, MPH, William D. Mosher, PhD. "Use of Infer-
      tility Services in the United States." *Obstetrics and Gynecology* vol. 82,
      no. 1 (July 1993): 123, 124.

39   Robin, *How to Be a Successful Fertility Patient*, p. 257.

40   "Against the Odds: How the Methods Compare." *Newsweek*. Septem-
      ber 4, 1995, p. 41.

41   Ibid.

42   Ibid.

43   Robin, *How to Be a Successful Fertility Patient*, p. 267.

44   Ibid., p. 271.

45   Ibid., p. 274.

46   Ibid., p. 282.

47   James P. Toner, MD, PhD, Jill Taylor Flood, MD. "Fertility After the
      Age of 40." *Obstetrics and Gynecology Clinics of North America* vol. 20,
      no. 1 (June 1993): 263. David B. Smotrich, MD, Eric A Widra, MD,
      Paul R. Gindoff, MD, Michael J. Levy, MD, Jerry L. Hall, PhD, Robert
      J. Stillman, MD. "Prognostic Value of Day 3 Estradiol on In Vitro
      Fertilization Outcome." *Fertility and Sterility* vol. 64, no. 6 (December
      1995): 1139.

48   Robin. *How to Be a Successful Fertility Patient*.

Chapter Five: Embracing Pregnancy Again

1   Kathleen Diamond, PhD. *Motherhood After Miscarriage*. Holbrook,
      Mass.: Bob Adams, Inc. 1991, p. 93.

2   Ibid., p. 102.

3   Dorothy Warburton, Jennie Kline, Zena Stein, Barbara Strobino. "Abnormalities in Spontaneous Abortions of Recognized Conceptions." *Perinatal Genetics: Diagnosis and Treatment.* Orlando, Florida: Academic Press, 1986, p. 36.

4   Diamond, *Motherhood After Miscarriage*, p. 138.

5   Ibid.

6   Diamond, *Motherhood After Miscarrage*.

7   Ibid., p. 173.

8   Ibid., p. 174.

9   Ibid., p. 209.

10 Ibid., p. 180.

11 Peggy Robin, *How to Be a Successful Fertility Patient.* New York: William Morrow, 1992, p. 221.

12 Diamond, *Motherhood After Miscarriage*, p. 180.

13 American Fertility Society. *A Guide for Patients.* Information sheet on hormonal abnormalities.

14 Diamond, *Motherhood After Miscarriage*, p. 188.

15 Boston Women's Health Book Collective. *The New Our Bodies, Ourselves.* New York: Simon and Schuster, 1992, p. 584.

16 Diamond, *Motherhood After Miscarriage*, p. 192.

17 Ibid., p. 194.

18 California Teratogen Information Service and Clinical Research Program. UCSD Medical Center, University of California, San Diego. Teratogen Information Specialist, 1/6/94, 8/7/96.

19 American Society of Reproductive Medicine (formerly American Fertility Society). *Recurrent Miscarriage: A Guide for Patients.* Patient information pamphlet. 1991, p. 7.

20 American College of Obstetricians and Gynecologists (ACOG), *Planning for Pregnancy, Birth and Beyond.* New York: Dutton, 1996, pp. 104, 105.

21 California Teratogen Information Service and Clinical Research Program. Teratogen Information Specialist. 1/6/94.

22 Ibid,. 1/6/94, 8/7/96.

23 Personal communication. Samuel Wood, MD, PhD. 12/23/96.

24 Diamond, *Motherhood After Miscarriage*, pp. 207, 208.

25 Ibid., p. 207.

26 Ibid., p. 144.

27 Personal communication. Deborah Wiseman, LVN. 3/24/97.

28 Personal communication. Samuel Wood, MD, PhD. 5/21/97.

29 Interview. William Hummel, MD. 2/23/94. Allen T. Bombard, MD, Robert W. Naef III, MD. "Reproductive Genetics for Couples Older Than 40 Years of Age." *Obstetrics and Gynecology Clinics of North America* vol. 20, no. 2 (June 1993): 289.

30 Ibid.

31 Ibid.

32 Bombard, Naef. "Reproductive Genetics for Couples Older Than 40," p. 289.

Chapter Six: Pregnancy Month by Month

1 George E. Verrilli, MD, FACOG, Anne Marie Mueser, EdD. *While Waiting: A Prenatal Guidebook.* New York: St. Martin's Press, 1989, p. 6.

2 *Mosby Medical Encyclopedia.* Revised edition. New York: Plume, 1992, p. 844.

3 Personal communication. Samuel Wood, MD, PhD. 12/10/96.

4 Sheila Kitzinger. *The Complete Book of Pregnancy and Childbirth.* New York: Knopf, 1986, p. 61.

5 *Mosby,* pp. 280, 611.

6 Kitzinger, *Complete Book of Pregnancy and Childbirth,* p. 62.

7 Verrilli, Mueser. *While Waiting: A Prenatal Guidebook,* p. 6.

8 Kathryn Schrotenboer-Cox, ob/gyn, Joan Solomon Weiss. *Pregnancy over 35.* New York. Ballantine Books, 1985, p. 48.

9   Ibid.

10   Ibid.

11   Health Education Associates, Inc. *Month by Month: How Your Baby Grows During Your Pregnancy.* Pamphlet. Sandwich, Mass. 1988, p. 3.

12   Janis Grahm, *Your Pregnancy Companion.* New York: Pocket Books, 1991, p. 12.

13   Kitzinger, *Complete Book of Pregnancy and Childbirth,* p. 322.

14   Kaiser Permanente, San Diego, Calif. Pregnancy test protocol. 1996.

15   Personal communication. Mayland Arrington, Clinical Laboratory Scientist, Owner, Claydelle Clinical Laboratory, El Cajon, Calif. 3/23/97.

16   *Mosby,* p. 627.

17   Ibid.

18   American College of Obstetricians and Gynecologists (ACOG). *Planning for Pregnancy, Birth and Beyond.* New York: Dutton, 1996, p. 52.

19   Ibid., pp. 50, 51.

20   Verrilli, Mueser, *While Waiting: A Prenatal Handbook.* p. 7.

21   Kitzinger, *Complete Book of Pregnancy and Childbirth,* p. 63.

22   Schrotenboer-Cox, Weiss, *Pregnancy over 35,* p. 48.

23   Health Education Associates, *Month by Month,* p. 3.

24   Grahm, *Your Pregnancy Companion,* p. 43.

25   Health Education Associates, *Month by Month,* p. 3.

26   Grahm, *Your Pregnancy Companion,* p. 43.

27   *Mosby,* p. 513.

28   Schrotenboer-Cox, Weiss, *Pregnancy over 35,* p. 29.

29   Margie Profet, *Protecting Your Baby-to-Be: Preventing Birth Defects in the First Trimester.* Reading, Mass.: Addison-Wesley, 1995, p. 99.

30   Miriam Erick, RD, MS. *No More Morning Sickness: A Survival Guide for Pregnant Women.* New York: Plume, 1993, p. 85.

31   Profet, *Protecting Your Baby-to-Be,* p. 196.

32   Ibid., pp. 8, 9, 99.

33   Ibid., pp. 8, 97, 98.

34   Kitzinger, *Complete Book of Pregnancy and Childbirth*, p. 325.

35   Erick, *No More Morning Sickness*, pp. 1, 5.

36   Ibid., p. 12.

37   Profet, *Protecting Your Baby-to-Be*, p. 194.

38   Erick, *No More Morning Sickness*, p. 5.

39   Profet, *Protecting Your Baby-to-Be*, p. 5.

40   Erick, *No More Morning Sickness*, p. 32.

41   Health Education Associates, *Month by Month*, p. 4.

42   Verrilli, Mueser. *While Waiting: A Prenatal Handbook*, p. 8.

43   Ibid.

44   Health Education Associates, *Month by Month*, p. 4.

45   Grahm, *Your Pregnancy Companion*, p. 64.

46   Verrilli, Mueser. *While Waiting: A Prenatal Handbook*, p. 8.

47   *Mosby*, p. 631.

48   Schrotenboer-Cox, Weiss. *Pregnancy over 35*, p. 49.

49   ACOG, *Planning for Pregnancy, Birth and Beyond*, p. 52.

50   *Mosby*, p. 630.

51   Ibid., p. 317. Profet, *Protecting Your Baby-to-Be*, pp. 1, 2.

52   Grahm, *Your Pregnancy Companion*, p. 64.

53   Kitzinger, *Complete Book of Pregnancy and Childbirth*, p. 324.

54   ACOG, *Planning for Pregnancy, Birth and Beyond*, p. 133.

55   Kitzinger, *Complete Book of Pregnancy and Childbirth*, p. 324.

56   Schrotenboer-Cox, Weiss. *Pregnancy over 35*, p. 29.

57   Interview. William Hummel, MD. 2/23/94. Allen T. Bombard, MD, Robert W. Naef III, MD. Reproductive Genetics for Couples Older Than 40 Years of Age. *Obstetrics and Gynecology Clinics of North America* vol. 20, no. 2 (June 1993): 289.

58   Childbirth Education Associates of San Diego (CEA of San Diego).

Preparing for Childbirth: Pregnancy-Birth-Postpartum. San Diego, 1986, p. 23.

59   Nancy F. Josephson, "What You May Not Know About Pregnancy Tests." *Parents.* April 1996, p. 78.

60   ACOG, *Planning for Pregnancy, Birth and Beyond,* p. 170.

61   Josephson, "What You May Not Know About Pregnancy Tests," p. 77.

62   Ibid. *Mosby,* p. 40.

63   Josephson, "What You May Not Know About Pregnancy Tests," p. 78.

64   ACOG, *Planning for Pregnancy, Birth and Beyond,* p. 187. *Mosby,* p. 744.

65   ACOG, *Planning for Pregnancy, Birth and Beyond,* p. 194.

66   Ibid., pp. 184, 185.

67   Ibid., p. 52.

68   *Mosby,* p. 688.

69   ACOG, *Planning for Pregnancy, Birth and Beyond,* p. 192.

70   Ibid.

71   Ibid., p. 52.

72   Josephson, "What You May Not Know About Pregnancy Tests," p. 78.

73   ACOG, *Planning for Pregnancy, Birth and Beyond,* p. 198.

74   Ibid. *Mosby,* p. 780.

75   ACOG, *Planning for Pregnancy, Birth and Beyond,* p. 198.

76   CEA of San Diego, *Preparing for Childbirth,* p. 23.

77   Kitzinger, *Complete Book of Pregnancy and Childbirth,* p. 121. ACOG, *Planning for Pregnancy, Birth and Beyond,* p. 154.

78   ACOG, *Planning for Pregnancy, Birth and Beyond,* p. 154.

79   Arlene Eisenberg, Heidi E. Murkoff, Sandee E. Hathaway, BSN. *What to Expect When You're Expecting.* Second edition. New York: Workman Publishing, 1991, p. 353.

80   ACOG, *Planning for Pregnancy, Birth and Beyond,* p. 154.

81   CEA of San Diego, *Preparing for Childbirth*, p. 23.

82   ACOG, *Planning for Pregnancy, Birth and Beyond*, p. 155.

83   Ibid., p. 49.

84   Personal communication. Deborah Wiseman, LVN. 12/20/96.

85   Personal communication. Gloria Anne Sanchez-Araiza, MS, MPH, Certified Genetics Counselor. 12/13/96.

86   ACOG, *Planning for Pregnancy, Birth and Beyond*, p. 53.

87   *Mosby*, p. 631.

88   Grahm, *Your Pregnancy Companion*, p. 87.

89   Health Education Associates, *Month by Month*, p. 6.

90   Ibid.

91   Verrilli, Mueser, *While Waiting: A Prenatal Guidebook*, p. 9.

92   Ibid.

93   Grahm, *Your Pregnancy Companion*, p. 86.

94   ACOG, *Planning for Pregnancy, Birth and Beyond*, p. 133.

95   Verrilli, Mueser, *While Waiting: A Prenatal Guidebook*, p. 17.

96   ACOG, *Planning for Pregnancy, Birth and Beyond*, p. 133.

97   Kitzinger, *Complete Book of Pregnancy and Childbirth*, p. 325.

98   *Mosby*, p. 628.

99   Ibid.

100 ACOG, *Planning for Pregnancy, Birth and Beyond*, p. 123, 124.

101 Ibid., pp. 126, 127.

102 Profet, *Protecting Your Baby-to-Be*, p. 189.

103 *Mosby*, p. 629. Interview. Janice Baker, RD, Certified Diabetes Educator. 2/25/94.

104 Schrotenboer-Cox, Weiss. *Pregnancy over 35*, p. 55.

105 Personal communication. Janice Baker, RD, Certified Diabetes Educator. 11/20/96. Dairy Council of California. *Pregnancy: A Special Time for Nutrition and Good Health*. Booklet. 10/91, p. 5.

106 ACOG, *Planning for Pregnancy, Birth and Beyond*, p. 123.

107 Grahm, *Your Pregnancy Companion*, pp. 54, 55.

108 ACOG. Preterm Labor. *Technical Bulletin* no. 206 (June 1995): 1, 8. *Mosby*, p. 472.

109 Baker, 2/25/94.

110 Ibid.

111 *Mosby*, p. 453.

112 Ibid., p. 819.

113 Health Education Associates, *Month by Month*, p. 7.

114 Ibid.

115 *Mosby*, p. 631.

116 Grahm, *Your Pregnancy Companion*, p. 100.

117 Ibid., p. 99.

118 Verrilli, Mueser, *While Waiting: A Prenatal Guidebook*, p. 17.

119 Kitzinger, *Complete Book of Pregnancy and Childbirth*, p. 31.

120 Schroenboer-Cox, Weiss, *Pregnancy over 35*, p. 44.

121 Grahm, *Your Pregnancy Companion*, p. 95.

122 *Mosby*, p. 655. ACOG, *Planning for Pregnancy, Birth and Beyond*, p. 52.

123 Schrotenboer-Cox, Weiss, *Pregnancy over 35*, p. 29.

124 ACOG, *Planning for Pregnancy, Birth and Beyond*, p. 136.

125 Ibid., p. 88.

126 Ibid.

127 Ibid., pp. 88–91. ACOG. "Exercise During Pregnancy and the Postpartum Period." *Technical Bulletin* no. 189 (February 1994). ACOG. *Exercise and Fitness: A Guide for Women*. Patient education pamphlet. December 1992.

128 ACOG, "Exercise during pregnancy and the postpartum period," p. 3.

129 Grahm, *Your Pregnancy Companion*, p. 111.

130 Health Education Associates, *Month by Month*, p. 8.

131 Ibid.

132 Ibid.

133 Ibid.

134 Kitzinger, *Complete Book of Pregnancy and Childbirth*, p. 328.

135 Grahm, *Pregnancy Companion*, p. 111.

136 Personal communication. Howard A. Schneider, MD, Director, Neonatal Intensive Care Unit, Kaiser Permanenete, San Diego Medical Center. San Diego, Calif. 12/19/96.

137 ACOG, "Preterm labor," p. 7.

138 Personal communication. Howard A. Schneider, MD, Director, Neonatal Intensive Care Unit, Kaiser Permanente, San Diego Medical Center. San Diego, Calif. 12/24/96.

139 ACOG, *Planning for Pregnancy, Birth and Beyond*, p. 179.

140 Ibid., p. 50.

141 *Mosby*, p. 627.

142 ACOG, *Planning for Pregnancy, Birth and Beyond*, pp. 179, 180.

143 Ibid., pp. 175, 179.

144 *Mosby*, p. 629.

145 ACOG, "Preterm Labor," p. 1.

146 March of Dimes. *Premature Labor: A Teaching Guide for Pregnant Women*. March of Dimes Birth Defects Foundation. White Plains, NY. February 1989, p. 2.

147 ACOG, "Preterm Labor," p. 7.

148 Ibid.

149 Schneider, 12/24/96.

150 Health Education Associates, *Month by Month*, p. 9.

151 Ibid.

152 Kitzinger, *Complete Book of Pregnancy and Childbirth*, p. 66.

153 Ibid.

154 Schrotenboer-Cox, Weiss, *Pregnancy over 35*, pp. 49, 50.

155 Health Education Associates, *Month by Month* p. 9.

156 Grahm, *Your Pregnancy Companion*, p. 127.

157 Kitzinger, *Complete Book of Pregnancy and Childbirth*, p. 329.

158 *Mosby*, p. 113.

159 Verrilli, Mueser, *While Waiting: A Prenatal Guidebook*, p. 17.

160 *Mosby*, p. 113.

161 Kitzinger, *Complete Book of Pregnancy and Childbirth*, p. 329. ACOG, *Planning for Pregnancy, Birth and Beyond*, p. 134.

162 CEA of San Diego, *Preparing for Childbirth*, p. 78.

163 Boston Women's Health Collective. *The New Our Bodies, Ourselves.* New York: Simon and Schuster, 1992, p. 478.

164 Ibid.

165 CEA of San Diego, *Preparing for Childbirth*, p. 78.

166 Kitzinger, *Complete Book of Pregnancy and Childbirth*, p. 67.

167 Ibid., p. 330.

168 Grahm, *Your Pregnancy Companion*, p. 144.

169 Verrilli, Mueser, *While Waiting: A Prenatal Guidebook*, p. 17.

170 Schneider, 12/24/96.

171 Kitzinger, *Complete Book of Pregnancy and Childbirth*, p. 331.

172 Eisenberg, et al. *What to Expect When You're Expecting*, p. 257.

173 Health Education Associates, *Month by Month*, p. 10.

174 *Mosby*, p. 631.

175 Health Education Associates, *Month by Month*, p. 10.

176 Ibid.

177 Grahm, *Your Pregnancy Companion*, p. 182.

178 ACOG, *Planning for Pregnancy, Birth and Beyond*, p. 134.

179 Ibid., p. 135.

180 Kitzinger, *Complete Book of Pregnancy and Childbirth*, p. 67.

181 ACOG, *Planning for Pregnancy, Birth and Beyond*, pp. 134, 135.

182 *Mosby*, p. 274. CEA of San Diego, *Preparing for Childbirth*, p. 29. Kitzinger, *Complete Book of Pregnancy and Childbirth*, p. 203.

183 Eisenberg, et al., *What to Expect When You're Expecting*, p. 261.

184 CEA of San Diego, *Preparing for Childbirth*, p. 32.

185 Ibid.

186 CEA of San Diego, *Preparing for Childbirth*, p. 33. ACOG, *Planning for Pregnancy, Birth and Beyond*, p. 208.

187 Kaiser Permanente. *Pregnancy: A New Beginning*. A prenatal guide for expectant parents. Southern California region. 1988, p. 60.

188 ACOG, *Planning for Pregnancy, Birth and Beyond*, p. 211.

189 Schrotenboer-Cox, Weiss, *Pregnancy over 35*, p. 177.

190 Ibid. pp. 177, 178. Verrilli, Mueser, *While Waiting: A Prenatal Guidebook*, p. 62.

191 Kitzinger, *Complete Book of Pregnancy and Childbirth*, p. 161. Verrilli, Mueser, *While Waiting: A Prenatal Guidebook*, p. 62.

192 CEA of San Diego, p. 53. ACOG, *Planning for Pregnancy, Birth and Beyond*, p. 222.

193 CEA of San Diego, p. 53. Eisenberg, et al. *What to Expect When You're Expecting*, p. 229.

194 ACOG, *Planning for Pregnancy, Birth and Beyond*, p. 224.

195 Ibid.

196 Ibid., pp. 225, 226.

197 Wood, 12/10/96.

Appendix A: Should I Worry? Potential Danger Signs During Pregnancy

1 American College of Obstetricians and Gynecologists (ACOG). *Planning for Pregnancy, Birth and Beyond*. New York: Dutton, 1996, p. 166.

2 Sheila Kitzinger. *The Complete Book of Pregnancy and Childbirth*. New York: Knopf, p. 120.

3 American Society for Reproductive Medicine (formerly American Fer-

tility Society). *Recurrent Miscarriage: A Guide for Patients.* Patient information pamphlet. 1991, p. 7.

4 *Mosby Medical Encyclopedia.* Revised edition. New York: Plume, 1992, p. 611.

5 Ibid.

6 Kitzinger, *Complete Book of Pregnancy and Childbirth,* p. 120.

7 Kaiser Permanente. *You Can Help You and Your Baby By Checking for Uterine Contractions.* Information sheet.

8 Ibid.

9 ACOG, *Planning for Pregnancy, Birth and Beyond,* p. 176.

10 ACOG, "Preterm Labor." *Technical Bulletin,* no. 206 (June 1995): p. 3. ACOG, *Planning for Pregnancy, Birth and Beyond,* p. 176.

11 Kaiser Permanente, *You Can Help You and Your Baby.*

12 ACOG, *Planning for Pregnancy, Birth and Beyond,* p. 176.

13 Kaiser Permanente, *You Can Help You and Your Baby.* March of Dimes, *Helpful Hints: Some Ideas to Help Prevent Preterm Labor.* White Plains, N.Y.: March of Dimes Birth Defects Foundation, 1992, p. 5.

14 Ibid.

15 March of Dimes, *Helpful Hints,* p. 5.

16 Ibid.

17 Kathryn Schrotenboer-Cox, ob/gyn, Joan Solomon Weiss. *Pregnancy over 35.* New York: Ballantine Books, 1985, pp. 40, 41.

18 ACOG, *Planning for Pregnancy, Birth and Beyond,* p. 60.

19 *Mosby,* p. 627. ACOG, *Planning for Pregnancy, Birth and Beyond,* p. 152.

20 Gertrud S. Berkowitz, PhD, Mary Louise Skovron, DrPh, Robert H. Lapinski, PhD, Richard L. Berkowitz, MD. "Delayed Childbearing and the Outcome of Pregnancy." *New England Journal of Medicine* vol. 322, no. 10 (March 8, 1990): 661. ACOG, *Planning for Pregnancy, Birth and Beyond,* p. 152.

21 ACOG, *Planning for Pregnancy, Birth and Beyond,* p. 152.

22 Ibid. Childbirth Education Associates of San Diego, Inc. (CEA of San Diego) *Pregnancy-Birth-Postpartum.* San Diego, Calif., 1986, p. 6.

Appendix B: Basic Food Guide: Preconception-Pregnancy-Nursing

1   American College of Obstetricians and Gynecologists (ACOG). *Planning for Pregnancy, Birth and Beyond.* New York: Dutton, 1996, p. 128.

2   Ibid.

3   Personal communication. Janice Baker, RD, Certified Diabetes Educator. 5/16/97.

4   Baker, 12/2/96.

5   Baker, 12/2/96, 5/16/97. ACOG, *Planning for Pregnancy, Birth and Beyond.* p. 119. "Dietary Guidelines Modified from the United States Department of Agriculture and United States Department of Health and Human Services." Dairy Council of California, *Pregnancy: A Special Time for Nutrition and Good Health.* 1993, p. 11. Kaiser Permanente, *Eating for Two, Nutrition for Pregnancy and Breast Feeding.* Health education pamphlet. Southern California region. 8/82.

6   Personal communication. Janice Baker, RD, Certified Diabetes Educator. 10/14/96. Baker, 5/16/97. ACOG, *Planning for Pregnancy, Birth and Beyond,* pp. 117–119. Kaiser Permanente, *Eating for Two.*

7   Ibid.

8   United States Department of Health and Human Services. (DHSS). "Recommendations for the Use of Folic Acid to Reduce the Number of Cases of Spina Bifida and Other Neural Tube Defects." *Center for Disease Control Morbidity and Mortality Weekly Report* vol. 41, no. RR-14 (September 11, 1992): 1, 5. Personal communication. Richard Olney, MD, MPH. Medical Epidemiologist, Center for Disease Control and Prevention. 12/17/96.

9   Food and Nutrition Board, Commission on Life Sciences, National Research Council, *Recommended Dietary Allowances.* Tenth edition. Washington, D.C.: National Academy Press, 1989, appendix.

10   Olney, 12/17/96. United States DHHS. "Recommendations for the Use of Folic Acid," p. 1.

11   ACOG, *Planning for Pregnancy, Birth and Beyond,* p. 76.

12   California Teratogen Information Service and Clinical Research Pro-

gram, UCSD Medical Center, University of California, San Diego. Teratogen Information Specialist, 5/18/96.

13 Baker, 12/2/96.

14 "Foodborne Illness: Role of Home Food Handling Practices." *Food Technology* vol. 49, no. 4 (April 1995): 122, 124. Reprinted from the American Council on Science and Health (ACSH), New York.

Index